Recent Advances in

Obstetrics & Gynaecology

26

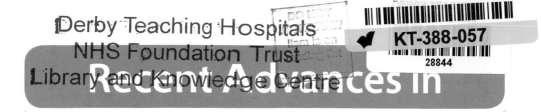

Recent Advances in

Obstetrics & Gynaecology
26

William Ledger MA DPhil Oxon MB ChB FRCOG FRANZCOG CREI
Professor of Obstetrics and Gynaecology
Royal Hospital for Women
Randwick, Australia

Justin Clark MD MRCOG
Department of Obstetrics and Gynaecology
Birmingham Women's Hospital
Birmingham, UK

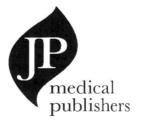

JP
medical
publishers

London • Philadelphia • Panama City • New Delhi

© 2015 JP Medical Ltd.
Published by JP Medical Ltd,
83 Victoria Street, London, SW1H 0HW, UK
Tel: +44 (0)20 3170 8910   Fax: +44 (0)20 3008 6180
Email: info@jpmedpub.com   Web: www.jpmedpub.com

ISBN: 978-1-909836-26-6

British Library Cataloguing in Publication Data
A catalogue record for this book is available from the British Library

Library of Congress Cataloging in Publication Data
A catalog record for this book is available from the Library of Congress

Commissioning Editor: Steffan Clements
Editorial Assistant: Sophie Woolven
Design: Designers Collective Ltd

Preface

In compiling this volume of *Recent Advances in Obstetrics & Gynaecology* we have combined authoritative reviews of relevance to all those with an interest in obstetrics and gynaecology with more specialist chapters that summarise progress in the most rapidly moving areas of our specialty.

We believe this mixture of general and specialist provides our readers with a broad overview of developments in the area, some of which may lie outside their daily practice but all of which we hope will be interesting and informative. In addition, many of our readers use *Recent Advances in Obstetrics & Gynaecology* to assist with exam revision and we are confident that this volume will not let them down.

The role of compilations of topical reviews such as this has been questioned: `what is the point of Recent Advances when limitless information can be accessed at the touch of a keyboard'? We believe the answer lies in the quality of these reviews and particularly in the quality of the authors, who provide an accessible and readable distillation of the complex evidence that surrounds the topics chosen for inclusion. We hope these give our readers the confidence of knowing they are up-to-date and have not missed any important developments in the field.

Limitless information demands limitless time for processing and who amongst us has such a luxury?

William Ledger
Justin Clark
July 2015

Contents

Contents

Chapter 1

Use of aortic balloon in massive postpartum haemorrhage

Roberto Brunelli

INTRODUCTION

Postpartum haemorrhage (PPH) remains a major cause of maternal mortality and severe morbidity. In the event of haemorrhage refractory to pharmacological intervention, obstetricians have traditionally resorted to hysterectomy. Over the past two decades, the treatment of PPH by interventional radiologists has provided a safe and effective alternative to surgery in many cases. Intravascular aortic balloon occlusion (IABO) has an emerging roll in the management of life-threatening PPH and in the conservative management of abnormal placentation.

IABO IN LIFE-THREATENING PPH

Primary post partum haemorrhage (pPPH) is defined as blood loss of over 500 mls in the 24 hours after delivery. Severe postpartum haemorrhage (sPPH) is a dramatic and life-threatening condition, variably defined as an estimated PPH ≥ 1800 mL (corresponding to a volume deficit of 30–35%) [1] or the presence of haemodynamic shock (defined by the need for continuous perfusion of vasopressors) with/without evidence of disseminated intravascular coagulation (DIC) [2].

The causes of pPPH include uterine atony (80% of cases), uterine and genital tract lacerations, retained products of conception, invasive placentation and coagulopathy. Available conservative options for pPPH include:
- pelvic arterial embolisation (PAE)
- balloon tamponade
- uterine compression sutures.

PAE is a highly effective procedure in controlling less severe pPPH, as confirmed by a recent meta-analysis showing an overall success rate of 90.7% [3]. However, current evidence suggests that balloon tamponade and uterine compression sutures must be considered as first-line treatments when pPPH results from uterine atony, with success rates of 84% and 91.7% respectively. These success rates are similar to those reported for PAE without the need for complex logistics [4].

Roberto Brunelli MD, Department of Gynecology Obstetrics and Urology, Università Sapienza, Roma, Italy. Email: roberto.brunelli@uniroma1.it (for correspondence)

However, PAE, balloon tamponade and uterine compression sutures can be dangerous in patients with sPPH because the success rate for PAE in patients with sPPH is much lower (71%) than that reported for less severe haemorrhage [2]. Also, balloon tamponade and uterine sutures may further worsen the compromised uterine blood supply, therefore increasing local lactic acid accumulation with an ultimate decrease in myometrial contractility [5].

The first priority in the management of patients with sPPH is haemodynamic stabilisation. This is the only clinical intervention that can allow for a safe primary hysterectomy or reasonable attempts at uterine preservation.

Clamping of the aorta has been performed since the beginning of aortic surgery and IABO is frequently employed to control profuse bleeding during hepato-pancreato-biliary surgery [6] or major pelvic surgical procedures [7].

Of note, aortic balloon occlusion grants a high degree of pelvic devascularisation and it is associated with important pathophysiologic modifications that counteract the progress of cardiocirculatory decompensation, including increased afterload with proximal arterial hypertension, increased end-diastolic ventricular volume with enhanced myocardial contractility and increased preload, resulting from blood volume redistribution from the veins distal to the aortic occlusion to the proximal vasculature [8].

Recently, Søvik et al reported the successful use of IABO in five patients with life-threatening PPH originating from uterine atonia [9]. In this emergency setting, IABO was performed directly in the operating room of the Department of Gynecology and Obstetrics by the on-call interventional radiologist without fluoroscopic guidance. IABO effectively improved the haemodynamic parameters of all patients with a reported mean increase of systolic blood pressure of 40 mmHg. The favourable clinical outcome observed in three patients who underwent primary hysterectomy was attributed both to a better view of the operating field and to the benefits of IABO circulatory effects. In two patients, IABO haemodynamic stabilisation provided time to allow effective treatment with uterotonic drugs, avoiding hysterectomy. The improvement in the patient's haemodynamic status caused by IABO may provide time to perform successful PAE. Patients selected for selective embolisation should therefore be transferred to the angiographic suite as soon as possible.

Extended use of IABO has been correlated with reduced survival rates in trauma patients with pelvic fractures and massive haemorrhage. This has been explained by the effects of the haemodynamic depression that occurs upon balloon deflation as a result of toxin release and worsening acidosis triggered by leg ischaemia [10]. Because of the risk of these ischaemic complications, the approach to sPPH reported by Søvik et al used a protocol of periodic deflation of the aortic balloon every 10–15 minutes that allowed both for evaluation of the amount of ongoing bleeding and for reperfusion of the lower limbs and occluded organs. Significantly, as noted by the authors, blind (non-fluoroscopic) IABO may have resulted in renal artery occlusion in some patients. However, it is known that the kidneys can withstand up to 40 minutes of warm ischaemia without damage [9]; so, this relatively brief period of possible renal artery occlusion was considered clinically irrelevant.

IABO IN CAESAREAN HYSTERECTOMY FOR PLACENTA PERCRETA

Abnormal placentation occurs when a defect within the decidua basalis allows invasion of chorionic villi into the myometrium. Placenta accreta, increta and percreta represent a spectrum of placental adhesive disorders marked by a progressively increasing invasion of the myometrium. The recommended treatment for placenta accreta is caesarean hysterectomy whilst leaving the placenta in situ, to avoid the massive bleeding that occurs upon placental disruption and may lead to severe morbidity and significant risk of death [11].

Interventional radiology can play an important role during caesarean hysterectomy for placenta accreta as it can decrease the severity of haemorrhage and improve the surgical field, allowing for a more controlled hysterectomy.

A search of different databases with the keywords 'balloon catheter', 'arterial embolisation', 'post-partum haemorrhage', 'caesarean hysterectomy' and 'placenta accreta' identified no randomised controlled trials and only five case-control studies that investigated whether endovascular balloons positioned in the internal iliac arteries (IIA) immediately before caesarean section might decrease blood loss during caesarean hysterectomy (**Table 1.1**). Three studies failed to demonstrate that IIA occlusion/embolisation has any role in decreasing blood loss or transfusion requirements [12–14]. The two trials that supported the use of this form of interventional radiology mainly reported positive results in cases of placenta percreta [15,16]. The report by Cali et al identified that the effectiveness of IIA balloon occlusion in reducing intraoperative blood loss was limited to cases of placenta percreta (corresponding to 13/23 and 18/30 cases in the control and treated group respectively) with no advantage being recorded for cases of placenta accreta/increta [15]. Similarly, the study by Tan et al [16] reported a high prevalence of placenta percreta (7/11 patients and 7/14 patients in the study and control groups respectively). Overall, evidence supporting an ancillary role for IIA occlusion/embolisation during caesarean hysterectomy is limited to cases of placenta percreta.

The sophisticated and costly equipment required for successful IIA catheterisation is not available in many operating rooms, and many radiology suites are either geographically distant from the operating room or do not conform to its standards. IIA occlusion/embolisation is complex to perform and carries risk of maternal thromboembolic events [17] and possible effects of fetal radiation exposure, albeit reduced in recent protocols that used short-time fluoroscopy (<5 minutes) [15,16].

Temporary cross-clamping of the infrarenal abdominal aorta during caesarean hysterectomy has been proposed as an effective method for control of bleeding in cases of severe invasive placentation [18]; however, surgical retroperitoneal dissection of the aorta is difficult and a wide application of this approach is unlikely.

Endovascular catheterisation of the aorta can have a similar effect to aortic cross-clamping, is less technically demanding than retroperitoneal dissection or IIA catheterisation, can be performed easily in the operating room as a blind procedure or with the help of a few seconds of fluoroscopy and is unlikely to affect the fetal circulation.

Case reports concerning the management of placenta percreta have described IABO as an emergency procedure used to manage acute intraoperative torrential bleeding [19,20] or as a prophylactic approach during scheduled caesarean hysterectomy [21,22].

IABO has recently been used in the department of gynecology, obstetrics and urology, in Università Sapienza, as part of the management of two patients with an ultrasound diagnosis of placenta percreta based on the evidence of a complete placenta praevia bulging into the urinary bladder with an absent hypoechoic retroplacental zone and multiple irregular lacunae. In both cases, elective caesarean hysterectomy under general anaesthesia was scheduled at 34 weeks. IABO was performed directly in the operating

Table 1.1 Summary of primary outcomes following balloon occlusion of the internal iliac arteries

Reference	N	IOL (mL)	Blood	Embolisation	HS	Complication related to the use of endovascular catheters
Dubois 1997 [31]	S = 2 C = 0	S = 1750	–	After balloon occlusion	8.5	–
Levine et al 1999 [12]	S = 5 C = 4	S = 5025 C = 4652	S = 5.5 U C = 4 U	–	S = 7 C = 5	–
Weeks 2000 [32]	S = 1 C = 0	S = 1500	S = 3 U	–	S = 8	–
Kidney 2001 [33]	S = 5 S = 0	S = 2240	S = 2.2 U	–		–
Ojala 2005 [34]	S = 7 C = 0	S = 4500	5.4 U	After balloon occlusion		–
Bodner and Nosher 2006 [13]	S = 6 C = 22	S = 2800 C = 2600	S = 6.5 U C = 6.3 U	After balloon occlusion	S = 6.2 C = 5.9	–
Tan et al 2007 [16]	S = 11 C = 14	S = 2011 C = 3316	S = 1058 mL C = 2211 mL	–	S = 6.7 C = 4.9	–
Greenberg 2007 [35]	S = 1 C = 0	S = 2000	S = 6 U	–	S = 4	Iliac artery thrombosis
Shrivastava et al 2007 [14]	S = 19 C = 50	S = 2700 C = 3000	S = 10 U C = 6.5 U	–	S = 5 C = 4	Three severe complication
Mok 2008 [36]	S = 13 C = 0	S = 6415	S = 12.9 U	–		Mild left leg claudication
Sivan et al 2010 [26]	S = 23 C = 0	S = 2000	–	After balloon occlusion	S = 8	One stent placement One arterial bypass
Carnevale 2011 [37]	S = 21 C = 0	S = 1671	S = 1.2 U	-		Two thromboembolectomy
Thon 2011 [38]	S = 14 C = 0	S = 4632	S = 4.3 U	–		One left groin haematoma Migration of catheters from internal iliac arteries
Bishop 2011 [39]	S = 0 C = 0	S = 15000		After complication		Bilateral pseudoaneurysm, Unilateral arterial rupture Compromised vascular supply to the right leg secondary to thrombus formation
Knuttien 2012 [40]	S = 1 C = 0	S = 4500	S = 4 U	–		–
Clausen 2012 [41]	S = 17 C = 0	S = 4050	1780 mL	–	S = 8	–
Teixidor 2014 [42]	S = 27 C = 0	S = 1920	Not available	After balloon occlusion	S = 6	One case of iliac artery thrombosis
Cali 2014 [15]	S = 30 C = 23	S = 933 C = 1507	S = 0.6 U C = 3.3 U	–	S = 7.0 C = 7.6	–

N, number of cases; S, study group; C, control group in which patients underwent hysterectomy alone; IOL, intraoperative blood loss; Blood, units of packed red cells or blood volumes without further specifications; HS, hospital stay (days).

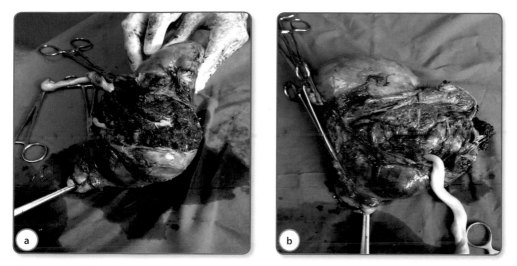

Figure 1.1a and b Intraoperative findings of placenta percreta.

room under local anaesthesia immediately before caesarean section. In order to reduce the diameter of the introducing sheaths, using a standard Seldinger technique, two 8-F occlusion balloons catheters were inserted between the iliac bifurcation and the renal arteries. The correct placement of the balloons was confirmed in both cases by fluoroscopy (<5 seconds) with an estimated fetal exposure of approximately 0.1 mGy. No abnormalities of the fetal heart rate were recorded during the entire procedure. Intraoperative confirmation of percreta was obtained for both patients (**Figure 1.1a** and **Figure 1.1b**) [11,12]. Upon cord clamping, the occlusion balloons were inflated to the size needed to occlude the aorta (3/4 mL of saline solution to a pressure of 810–1013 kPa); Doppler assessment of the common femoral artery recorded a residual blood flow of 10–15%. In the two patients, the estimated blood losses (EBLs), measured with reference to the contents of the suction jar and to the weight of the surgical pads at the end of surgery, were 830 and 945 mL respectively. This blood loss originated almost completely from marked oozing in the pelvic cavity that occurred after balloon deflation at the end of the hysterectomy. Notably, patients received no blood products.

The significance of the present evidence is obviously hampered by the absence of a control group; however, the results are similar, in terms of blood loss and absence of need for blood products, to those obtained by Cali et al using IIA occlusion [19]. Further research is needed, with reports from other centres, before IABO should be regarded as the ancillary procedure of choice during scheduled caesarean hysterectomy for placenta percreta but IABO seems to offer a safe and simple means or reducing blood loss in such cases.

IABO AND PRESERVATION OF FERTILITY IN CASES OF PLACENTA ACCRETA

The use of elective hysterectomy for placenta accreta is an unacceptable for women who wish to preserve their fertility. In these cases, uterine preservation can be attempted by leaving the placenta in place without any manual manipulation.

The largest multicentre study of this type of conservative surgery was reported by Sentilhes et al [23]. In this report, the overall success rate in 167 cases of placenta accreta undergoing conservative treatment leaving the placenta in situ was 78.4%, with a severe maternal morbidity rate of 6.0%. Thirty-six women had an unfavourable outcome: 18 underwent primary hysterectomy for primary PPH (i.e. within the first 24 hours after delivery), whilst 18 delayed hysterectomies were prompted by different complications including secondary haemorrhage (8/18), sepsis (2/18), secondary haemorrhage with sepsis (2/18), uterine necrosis and sepsis (2/18), vesicouterine fistula (1/18), arteriovenous malformation (1/18) and maternal request (1/18). Spontaneous placental resorption occurred with a median delay of 13.5 weeks from delivery (range 4–60 weeks).

The possible complications of placental retention and the need for long-term follow-up are unacceptable for some women who wish to try to conceive again, particularly those who are already older than 30 years. Extirpative management of the placenta with resection of the invaded area has been recommended for this group of patients but this procedure carries a high risk of severe intraoperative haemorrhage, ultimately leading to hysterectomy in a significant proportion of cases [24]. The outcome of the conservative/extirpative approach can be improved by temporary pelvic devascularisation, allowing the surgeon to curette and oversew the placental implantation site with an acceptable blood loss. As previously mentioned, the available evidence does not support IIA occlusion as an effective approach to reduce the extent of haemorrhage during caesarean hysterectomy for placenta accreta/increta and therefore this technique does not appear to be a reasonable choice to increase the chances of uterine preservation if manual removal of morbidly adherent placenta is attempted.

IABO has been used by the department of gynecology, obstetrics and urology, in Università Sapienza, to decrease the hysterectomy rate in a group of patients desiring to preserve their fertility, who did not accept a conservative approach leaving the placenta in situ and who received an ultrasound diagnosis (confirmed at MRI) of placenta praevia multifocally accreta (i.e. at least two evident disruptions of the placenta–myometrium interface) or increta [25]. For all patients, the diagnosis was confirmed histologically from biopsies or hysterectomy specimens or by the intraoperative finding of a difficult placental separation followed by a heavy bleeding from the implantation site. Scheduled caesarean delivery was performed at 36 weeks ±2 days gestation. The technical approach to IABO was as described in the previous section of this chapter regarding its use during caesarean hysterectomy. The occlusion balloons were inflated soon after cord clamping and deflated after achieving an effective haemostasis.

In 33 consecutive and comparable patients (based on demographics, history of caesarean section and incidence of multifocal accreta/increta), the placenta was systematically removed and control of bleeding from the implantation site was attempted by oversewing of the implantation site and/or performing a lower uterine curettage. Hysterectomy was started if these procedures did not arrest profuse bleeding or when the EBL was $\geq$1800 mL (grade 3 haemorrhage). Overall, 15 patients were treated with IABO and 18 entered the control group according to their acceptance or refusal of the proposed IABO. Mean occlusion time was 32 minutes (range 25–39 minutes).

The hysterectomy rate in the IABO group was significantly lower than that in the control group (13% vs. 50%) ($P < 0.034$) and only 1/13 patients with multifocal accreta required hysterectomy (7%). EBL was 950 mL and 3375 mL in the IABO and control groups ($P < 0.001$). Coagulation disorders were not recorded in the IABO group and were present in 3/18 patients in the control group (16%); this difference was not significant, probably because of the small sample size.

No complications resulted from the placement of the aortic balloon and no patient suffered from reperfusion injury. IABO did not affect the fetal–placental circulation and no abnormalities of the fetal heart rate were recorded during the procedure, with Apgar scores at 5 minutes of >8 for all delivered fetuses.

There is only one other study that has reported experience of IABO in this setting. This study described a similarly low hysterectomy rate (8%) during extirpative management of placenta accreta [26]. However, in this report, the median blood loss (2000 mL) and incidence of DIC (24%) were both much higher than those reported for our patients, possibly reflecting the choice of these authors to use IIA occlusion/embolisation to complete surgery. Moreover, a critical evaluation of this report is hampered by the absence of a control group and by the uncertain histopathology of the presented cases. Indeed, MRI confirmation of the sonographic diagnosis of placenta accreta was obtained in only 16% of patients, despite a reported intraoperative diagnosis of placenta percreta in 13/23 cases (52%).

The reduction in blood loss that follows use of IABO during an extirpative approach to placenta accreta/increta is superior to the results of alternative techniques such as PAE and uterine balloon tamponade. PAE greatly reduces the risk of primary haemorrhage during conservative management leaving the placenta in situ, but its use during extirpative surgery is far less conclusive with high failure rates being reported recently [27]. This finding fits with the basic physiological consideration that removal of the placenta accreta opens up large-calibre spiral vessels and sinuses that cannot be sealed by the embolising agent. Moreover, cases of placenta accreta are frequently preferentially embolised with the use of polyvinyl alcohol (PVA) particles increasing the risk of uterine necrosis [27].

Balloon tamponade is a very effective in the treatment of PPH due to uterine atony or placenta praevia, but is an unsuitable choice to attempt uterine preservation in the presence of placenta accreta/increta [28]. Nine cases of placenta accreta were conservatively managed by a protocol combining B-Lynch compression suture, Bakri balloon tamponade, multiple endouterine square haemostatic sutures and prophylactic catheterisation of the descending aorta without balloon inflation. The mean EBL was 1620 mL and one patient experienced overt haemodynamic instability [29]. The studies described above suggest that when attempting uterine preservation, inflating the aortic balloon soon after cord clamping together with a limited uterine manipulation is a more rational and effective approach as it limits blood loss, haemodynamic shock/coagulation disorders and the risk of uterine necrosis. This latter complication can be driven by myometrial hypoperfusion/lacerations, resulting from the contemporary outward and inward compressions exerted by the balloon and B-Lynch suture respectively [30].

CONCLUSION

The evidence presented in this chapter suggests that in pregnant patients, IABO is both minimally invasive and safe. The putative risks of aortic rupture, plaque dislodgement and reperfusion injury are unlikely to occur, given the short perfusion time. The procedure can easily be performed as a blind procedure or with the help of a very short fluoroscopy directly in the operating room with no need for complex logistics. In addition, IABO produces a high degree of pelvic devascularisation together with positive cardiocirculatory effects. IABO may emerge as a valuable life-saving procedure during severe peripartum haemorrhage and is a suitable method in the management of patients with abnormal placentation who desire preservation of fertility but prefer a single-time surgical approach.

Key points for clinical practice

- IABO is safe and minimally invasive. It can be easily performed in the operating room without complex logistics.
- IABO helps manage patients with abnormal placentation who desire preservation of fertility, but deny the risks of conservative management based on placental retention.
- IABO is a valuable ancillary procedure during scheduled caesarean hysterectomy for placenta percreta, as it greatly reduces blood loss.
- IABO produces a high degree of pelvic devascularisation together with positive cardiocirculatory effects; therefore, it can be considered as a life-saving procedure in cases of catastrophic peripartum haemorrhage.

REFERENCES

1. Francois KE, Foley MR. Antepartum and postpartum hemorrhage. In: Gabbe SG, Niebyl JR, Simpson JL, (eds), Obstetrics. Normal and problem pregnacies, 6th edition. Philadelphia; Elsevier Churchill Livingstone, 2012:415–444.
2. Touboul C, Badiou W, Pelage JP, et al. Efficacy of selective arterial embolisation for the treatment of life-threatening post-partum haemorrhage in a large population. PLoS One 2008; 3(11):e3819.
3. Doumouchtsis SK, Papageorghiou AT, Arulkumaran A, et al. Systematic review of conservative management of postpartum hemorrhage: what to do when medical treatment fails. Obstetr Gynecol Surv 2007; 62:540–547.
4. Royal College of Obstetricians and Gynaecologists (RCOG). Postpartum haemorrhage, prevention and management (green-top guide no. 52). London; RCOG, 2009.
5. Quenby S, Pierce SJ, Brigham S, et al. Dysfunctional labor and myometrial lactic acidosis. Obstet Gynecol 2004; 103:718–723.
6. Miura F, Takada T, Ochiai T, et al. Aortic occlusion balloon catheter technique is useful for uncontrollable massive intraabdominal bleeding after hepato-pancreato-biliary surgery. J Gastrointest Surg 2006; 10:519–522.
7. Yang L, Chong-Qi T, Hai-Bo S, et al. Appling the abdominal aortic-balloon occluding combine with blood pressure sensor of dorsal artery of foot to control bleeding during the pelvic and sacrum tumors surgery. J Surg Oncol 2008; 97:626–628.
8. Gelman S. The pathophysiology of aortic cross-clamping and unclamping. Anesthesiology 1995; 82:1026–1057.
9. Søvik E, Stokkeland P, Storm BS, et al. The use of aortic occlusion balloon catheter without fluoroscopy for life-threatening post-partum haemorrhage. Acta Anaesthesiol Scand 2012; 56:388–393.
10. Martinelli T, Thony F, Decléty P, et al. Intra-aortic balloon occlusion to salvage patients with life-threatening hemorrhagic shocks from pelvic fractures. J Trauma 2010; 68:942–948.
11. ACOG Practice Bulletin: Clinical Management Guidelines for Obstetrician-Gynecologists Number 76, October 2006: postpartum hemorrhage. Obstet Gynecol 2006; 108:1039–1047.
12. Levine AB, Kuhlman K, Bonn J. Placenta accreta: comparison of cases managed with and without pelvic artery balloon catheters. J Matern Fetal Med 1999; 8:173–176.
13. Bodner LJ, Nosher JL, Gribbin C, et al. Balloon-assisted occlusion of the internal iliac arteries in patients with placenta accrete/percreta. Cardiovasc Intervent Radiol 2006; 29:354–356.
14. Shrivastava V, Nageotte M, Major C, et al. Case control comparison of cesarean hysterectomy with and without prophylactic placement of intravascular balloon catheters for placenta accreta. Am J Obstet Gynecol 2007; 197:402, e1e5.
15. Cali G, Forlani F, Giambanco L, et al. Prophylactic use of intravascular balloon catheters in women with placenta accreta, increta and percreta. Eur J Obstet Gynecol Reprod Biol 2014; 179:36–41.
16. Tan CH, Tay KH, Sheah K. Perioperative endovascular internal iliac occlusion balloon placement in management of placenta accreta. Am J Roentgenol 2007; 189:1158–1163.
17. Heidemann B. Interventional radiology in the treatment of morbidly adherent placenta: are we asking the right questions? Int J Obstet Anesth 2011; 20:279–281.

18. Min-Min C, Yu-Min K, Huey-Chun W, et al. Temporary cross clamping of the infrarenal aorta during caesarean hysterecromy to control operative loss in placenta praevia increta/percreta. Taiwan J Obstet Gynecol 2010; 49:72–76.
19. Usman N, Noblet J, Low D, et al. Intra-aortic balloon occlusion without fluoroscopy for severe postpartum haemorrhage secondary to placenta percreta. Int J Obstet Anesth 2014; 23:91–93.
20. Bell-Thomas SM, Penketh RJ, Lord RH, et al. Emergency use of a transfemoral aortic occlusion catheter to control massive haemorrhage at caesarean hysterectomy. BJOG 2003; 110:1120–1122.
21. Masamoto H, Uehara H, Gibo M, et al. Elective use of aortic balloon occlusion in cesarean hysterectomy for placenta previa percreta. Gynecol Obstet Invest 2009; 67:92–95.
22. Paull JD, Smith J, Williams L, et al. Balloon occlusion of the abdominal aorta during caesarean hysterectomy for placenta percreta. Anaesth Intensive Care 1995; 23:731–734.
23. Sentilhes L, Ambroselli C, Kayem G, et al. Maternal outcome after conservative treatment of placenta accreta. Obstet Gynecol 2010; 115:526–534.
24. Mazouni C, Palacios-Jaraquemada JM, Deter R, et al. Differences in the management of suspected cases of placenta accreta in France and Argentina. Int J Gynaecol Obstet 2009; 107:1–3.
25. Panici PB, Anceschi M, Borgia ML, et al. Intraoperative aorta balloon occlusion: fertility preservation in patients with placenta previa accreta/increta. J Matern Fetal Neonatal Med 2012; 25:2512–2516.
26. Sivan E, Spira M, Achiron R, et al. Prophylactic pelvic artery catheterization and embolization in women with placenta accreta: can it prevent cesarean hysterectomy? Am J Perinatol 2010; 27:455–461.
27. Poujade O, Zappa M, Letendre I, et al. Predictive factors for failure of pelvic arterial embolization for postpartum hemorrhage. Int J Gynaecol Obstet 2012; 117:119–123.
28. Kumru P, Demirci O, Erdogdu E, et al. The Bakri balloon for the management of postpartum hemorrhage in cases with placenta previa. Eur J Obstet Gynecol Reprod Biol. 2013; 167:167–170.
29. Arduini M, Epicoco G, Clerici G, et al. B-Lynch suture, intrauterine balloon, and endouterine hemostatic suture for the management of postpartum hemorrhage due to placenta previa accreta. Int J Gynaecol Obstet 2010; 108:191–193.
30. Saman Kumara YV, Marasinghe JP, Condous GS, et al. Pregnancy complicated by a uterine fundal defect resultimg from a previous B-Lynch suture. BJOG 2009; 116:1815–1817.
31. Dubois J1, Garel L, Grignon A, et al. Placenta percreta: balloon occlusion and embolization of the internal iliac arteries to reduce intraoperative blood losses. Am J Obstet Gynecol 1997;176(3):723-6.
32. Weeks SM1, Stroud TH, Sandhu J, et al. Temporary balloon occlusion of the internal iliac arteries for control of hemorrhage during cesarean hysterectomy in a patient with placenta previa and placenta increta. J Vasc Interv Radiol 2000;11(5):622-4.
33. Kidney DD1, Nguyen AM, Ahdoot D, et al. Prophylactic perioperative hypogastric artery balloon occlusion in abnormal placentation. AJR Am J Roentgenol 2001;176(6):1521-4.
34. Ojala K, Perälä J, Kariniemi J, et al. Arterial embolization and prophylactic catheterization for the treatment for severe obstetric haemorrhage Acta Obstet Gynecol Scand 2005;84(11):1075-80.
35. Greenberg JI1, Suliman A, Iranpour P, et al. Prophylactic balloon occlusion of the internal iliac arteries to treat abnormal placentation: a cautionary case. Am J Obstet Gynecol 2007;197(5):470.e1-4.
36. Mok M1, Heidemann B, Dundas K, et al. Interventional radiology in women with suspected placenta accreta undergoing caesarean section. Int J Obstet Anesth 2008;17(3):255-61.
37. Carnevale FC1, Kondo MM, de Oliveira Sousa W Jr, et al. Perioperative temporary occlusion of the internal iliac arteries as prophylaxis in cesarean section at risk of hemorrhage in placenta accreta. Cardiovasc Intervent Radiol 2011;34(4):758-64.
38. Thon S1, McLintic A, Wagner Y. Prophylactic endovascular placement of internal iliac occlusion balloon catheters in parturients with placenta accreta: a retrospective case series. Int J Obstet Anesth 2011;20(1):64-70
39. Bishop S1, Butler K, Monaghan S, et al. Multiple complications following the use of prophylactic internal iliac artery balloon catheterisation in a patient with placenta percreta. Int J Obstet Anesth 2011;20(1):70-3.
40. Knuttinen MG1, Jani A, Gaba RC, et al. Balloon occlusion of the hypogastric arteries in the management of placenta accreta: a case report and review of the literature. Semin Intervent Radiol 2012;29(3):161-8.
41. Clausen C1, Stensballe J, Albrechtsen CK, et al. Balloon occlusion of the internal iliac arteries in the multidisciplinary management of placenta percreta. Acta Obstet Gynecol Scand 2013;92(4):386-91
42. Teixidor Viñas M1, Belli A, Arulkumaran S, et al. Prevention of postpartum haemorrhage and hysterectomy in patients with Morbidly Adherent Placenta: A cohort study comparing outcomes before and after introduction of the Triple-P procedure. Ultrasound Obstet Gynecol 2014;17 [Epub ahead of print].

Chapter 2

Fetal fibronectin and cervical ultrasound in prediction of preterm labour

Sarah J Stock, Jane E Norman

INTRODUCTION

Preterm birth is defined as delivery of a baby before 37 weeks' gestation. Globally, 15 million births are preterm each year, resulting in 1 million deaths [1]. Children born after preterm labour often have lifelong problems, and care results in a substantial economic burden such thatin the UK, the cost of preterm birth to the public sector is estimated at >£2.9 million [2].

The majority of preterm birth is spontaneous, i.e. preceded by either the spontaneous onset of contractions or spontaneous rupture of membranes. A UK population database study found that more than three quarters of singleton preterm births were spontaneous, preceded by preterm labour in 62% of cases or prelabour rupture of membranes in15% cases [3]. The remainder of cases were medically indicated preterm deliveries due to maternal or fetal complications.

Reducing morbidity and mortality associated with preterm birth is one of the biggest challenges in obstetrics. Improvement can only be achieved if obstetricians can reliably identify women at risk of preterm labour, allowing for timely intervention [4]. The ideal predictive test for preterm delivery should have sufficient sensitivity and specificity to ensure identification of women who will benefit from treatments for preterm labour, whilst avoiding unnecessary, and potential harmful treatment of women who will not deliver early or for whom such treatments would be ineffective.

POTENTIAL BENEFITS OF PREDICTION OF PRETERM LABOUR

There are two clinical situations where accurate prediction of spontaneous preterm birth can allow interventions that benefit babies. First, prediction before the onset of symptoms

Sarah J Stock MBChB PhD, MRC Centre for Reproductive Health, Queen's Medical Research Institute, Edinburgh, UK.
Email: sarah.stock@ed.ac.uk (for correspondence)

Jane E Norman MD FRCOG FRCPE FMedSci, MRC Centre for Reproductive Health, Queen's Medical Research Institute, Edinburgh, UK

of preterm labour can allow prophylactic treatments such as progesterone, cervical cerclage or cervical pessary to be given. These have been shown to decrease the incidence of preterm labour, although there is still limited evidence that they improve neonatal or longer term outcomes [5–7]. Second, prediction of preterm birth in women with signs and symptoms suggestive of preterm labour allows administration of antenatal steroids [8] and magnesium sulphate [9], each of which has been proved to reduce neonatal morbidity and mortality. It also facilitates arrangement of delivery in a unit with appropriate neonatal care facilities, which is beneficial [10]. Tocolytics may be given to allow time for maternal transfer, and for steroids and magnesium sulphate to become effective, although evidence of benefit for babies is again lacking [11].

A major benefit that results from accurate prediction of preterm birth is the avoidance of unnecessary, and potentially harmful, treatments. Treatments for preterm labour are not innocuous. Infection, uterine bleeding and preterm contractions have been associated with cervical cerclage placement [6] and although progesterone is thought to be safe, long-term follow-up data is not yet available [5]. If preterm labour has been wrongly diagnosed in women with symptoms of preterm labour, and delivery does not occur, steroids may also have adverse long-term consequences for the baby, especially if multiple courses are given. Magnesium sulphate is safe only within a narrow dosage range, and overdose can cause respiratory depression and cardiac arrest in the mother. Tocolytic therapy, even when appropriate, can have serious side effects for both mother and baby. Unnecessary interventions also result in significant costs to health services and families. Hospital admission and interhospital transfer have considerable economic implications and can be associated with significant problems for women and their families due to physical separation, emotional stress and financial burden.

EFFICACY OF OTHER PREDICTORS OF PRETERM BIRTH

A large number of biomarkers have been explored as predictors of increased risk of spontaneous preterm birth, including biochemical markers in blood, urine, cervical secretions and amniotic fluid, as well as ultrasound-based tests. However, few have been found to be potentially useful in the prediction and diagnosis of preterm labour. The potential value of a diagnostic test can be assessed by calculating its 'likelihood ratio', which is calculated from sensitivity and specificity and gives an idea of how likely it is that test results usefully change the probability that a condition is present or absent (**Table 2.1**). A test

Table 2.1 A guide to interpretation of test accuracy			
Category of test usefulness	Likelihood ratio for a positive test result	Likelihood for a negative test result	Interpretation
Very useful	>10	<0.1	Likely to generate large and often conclusive changes from pre-test to post-test probabilities
Useful	5–10	0.1–0.2	Likely to generate moderate shifts in pre-test to post-test probabilities
May be useful	2–5	0.2–0.5	Likely to generate small but sometimes important changes in pre-test to post-test probabilities
Not useful	1–2	0.5–1	May alter pre-test to post-test probabilities to a small (and rarely important) degree
Adapted from Honest et al (2009).			

with a positive likelihood ratio (LR) of >10 or a negative LR of <0.1 is likely to be very useful, whilst positive LRs >5 and negative LRs <0.2 are likely to provide some useful information. LRs outwith these levels are unlikely to provide useful diagnostic or prognostic information.

A comprehensive systematic review of potential predictors of preterm birth evaluated 22 different tests [12]. In general, the quality of the studies was poor, and no test had both good positive and negative LRs. Cervical length ultrasound and fetal fibronectin (fFN) were amongst the best performing tests, with LRs >5 in asymptomatic women, for delivery before 34 weeks. Cervical length also had an LR+ of >5 in symptomatic women for delivery before 34 weeks, whilst fFN had an LR of <0.2 in symptomatic women, indicating its potential in ruling out preterm labour. Other meta-analyses have indicated broadly similar test performances [13–15A]. Although their usefulness is moderate, they are the most commonly used tests in clinical practice in the UK [15B] and subsequent reviews have not identified any other markers that perform better than cervical length or fFN.

BIOLOGICAL BASIS AND MEASUREMENT OF CERVICAL LENGTH AND FFN AS PREDICTORS OF PRETERM LABOUR

Several different pathological processes cause preterm labour, including uterine stretch, congenital or acquired cervical insufficiency, decidual haemorrhage, infection and inflammation. Whatever the underlying cause, the result is cervical ripening and fetal membrane disruption, and these processes can start some weeks before delivery. Detection of these very early features of preterm labour is the basis of both cervical length and fFN testing. In asymptomatic women, the aim is to identify that the process of labour has silently begun. In symptomatic women, lack of evidence that these processes have started indicates impending preterm delivery is unlikely.

Cervical length

Cervical effacement is a crucial step in the process of parturition and studies have suggested that it can precede labour by many weeks. Cervical effacement and shortening progresses distally from the internal cervical os; thus, it can be seen on ultrasound before it can be detected on inspection or digital vaginal examination. The shorter the cervical length, the higher the likelihood of spontaneous preterm birth [12], with the risk being highest the earlier cervical shortening is detected.

Cervical length usually remains constant between 14 and 28 weeks' gestation. Measurements vary with study method, but in general, cervical length at this stage is normally distributed with the 50th centile around 35 mm, the 10th centile at 25 mm and the 5th centile at 20 mm [16]. There is a progressive decrease in cervical length in the third trimester. Parity, ethnicity and maternal height do not significantly influence cervical length, but values are likely to differ in singleton and multiple pregnancies [17].

Although there is a consistent association between cervical length below the 10th percentile (25 mm) and spontaneous preterm birth, there is no cut-off below which preterm delivery is inevitable. In a large prospective study of predictors of preterm labour, only 18% of women with cervical length <25 mm at 24 weeks of gestation delivered <35 weeks' gestation, even in the absence of any preventative treatment, and only 50% of women with a cervical length <13 mm (1st centile) delivered <35 weeks [16].

Reproducibility of any diagnostic test is important, and ultrasound-based tests are particularly liable to variation due to inter- and intraobserver variation if not performed rigorously. Standard procedures for cervical length measurement should be used to minimise subjective assessment and error, and false-positive and negative findings (**Figure 2.1**). The gold standard method for cervical length measurement uses transvaginal ultrasound. Transabdominal ultrasound is less reliable, as there is decreased resolution, fetal parts can obscure visualisation of the internal os and bladder filling can elongate the cervix [18]. Transperineal ultrasound has also been proposed, but it appears to be more difficult than transvaginal ultrasound and less reproducible [19].

Cervical length scanning is dependent on the availability of an appropriate ultrasound machine, and trained personnel. Online training programmes for transvaginal ultrasound assessment of cervical length are available from the Fetal Medicine Foundation and the Perinatal Quality Foundation, with the option of review of scans for accreditation. This should be encouraged to ensure standardised practice.

Fetal fibronectin

fFN is a large molecular weight (450 kD) extracellular matrix glycoprotein, which is thought to promote cellular adhesion at the placental and decidual chorionic interfaces. It is not normally present in cervical secretions between 22 and 35 weeks' gestational age. However, it is released in the cervical secretions when the extracellular matrix of the chorionic–decidual interface is disrupted in early labour. The concentration of fFN and the risk of preterm labour are linearly related [20].

fFN is available as a commercial test (Hologic). It is licensed for use between 22 and 35 weeks' gestation. The manufacturers do not recommend testing in women who have moderate or severe vaginal bleeding, cervical dilatation ≥3 cm or confirmed rupture of membranes. Sexual intercourse, vaginal examination or transvaginal ultrasound in the preceding 24 hours can increase the likelihood of false-positive results. Samples for fibronectin testing are usually taken at speculum examination, with a swab lightly

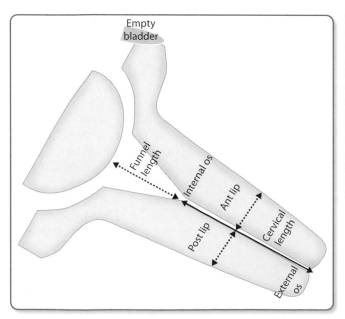

Figure 2.1 Cervical length measurement should be obtained by transvaginal scan with image filling approximately 75% of screen. The bladder should be empty, and the anterior and posterior lips of cervix should be of equal width in the image. The cervical length should be recorded as the length between internal and external os (thick black arrow). The dotted arrow is the funnel length, which should not be included in the cervical length measurement.

rotated across the posterior fornix of the vagina. Samples are analysed by a solid-phase immunochromatographic assay that uses murine monoclonal anti-fFN antibody conjugated to blue microspheres.

Originally, samples were read visually, similar to a pregnancy test, with test and control lines. A positive test line was seen if the concentration of fFN was 50 ng/mL or more. More recently, the test has been developed as a 'cassette', interpreted by a bedside analyser. The analyser has the advantages of internal quality controls, objective interpretation of results and a printed result with records stored for audit purposes. Results were again provided as POSITIVE or NEGATIVE on the basis of a single threshold of 50 ng/mL. Nearly all studies of fFN have been done based on this threshold. However, there are potential drawbacks to a qualitative diagnostic test based on a single threshold value. First, the test is prone to increased false-positive and negative tests around the cut-off point, and second, a qualitative test masks the improved prognostic ability of fibronectin levels at the extremes of the detection range. The newest version of the bedside analyser provides a concentration of fFN. The concentration of fibronectin may be a better predictor of outcome, although optimal thresholds for test use have not been fully validated.

The fFN system is designed to be an easy-to-perform point-of-care test. All reagents for fFN testing can be stored at room temperature and specimen collection kits, reagents, cassettes and the analyser can be kept in clinical areas where women with symptoms of preterm labour are assessed. The cost is approximately £40 per test.

PREDICTION OF PRETERM LABOUR IN ASYMPTOMATIC WOMEN

Cervical length as a predictor of preterm birth in asymptomatic women

In a recent meta-analysis of 23 studies of cervical length in asymptomatic women [15A], cervical length performed best when it was used to predict preterm birth <35 weeks gestation, and a cut off of 20mm was used. In these circumstances, the positive LR was 12.4 and the negative LR 0.74 (nine studies).

Fibronectin as a predictor of preterm birth in asymptomatic women

In the systematic review by Honest et al [12], the summary positive and negative LRs for delivery before 34 weeks' gestation were 7.65 [95% confidence interval (CI) 3.93–14.86] and 0.80 (95% CI 0.73–0.88). All studies used a threshold of 50 ng/mL and reported presence or absence of fibronectin. The new quantitative fFN analysers, which provide a concentration of fFN rather than a qualitative result (positive or negative) based on a single threshold, have shown promise as an improved predictor of spontaneous preterm birth. The concentration of fibronectin is correlated with the likelihood of delivery [20] and as a qualitative test based around a single threshold, important information regarding risk and fFN concentration may be missed. The EQUIPP study [21], a prospective masked observational study (n = 1448) of quantitative fFN testing in asymptomatic women at high risk of preterm birth between 22+0 and 27+6 weeks' gestation at five UK centres has recently been published [21]. The positive predictive value for spontaneous preterm birth at

<34 weeks' gestation was 37.7 (95% confidence interval 26.9–49.4), with a sensitivity of 46.7 (95% CI 31.7–62.1) and a specificity of 96% (95% CI 95.3–97.3) at a threshold of 200ng/ml. A fetal fibronectin concentration of less than 10 ng/mL was associated with a low risk of spontaneous preterm birth <34 weeks of gestation (2.7%).

Screening and treatment approaches in asymptomatic women

The potential ability of cervical length and fFN to predict spontaneous preterm birth in asymptomatic women has led them to be used in trials of treatments to prevent preterm labour. These have been performed in all maternities ('universal screening') or just selected women, though to be at high risk of spontaneous preterm birth based on clinical history.

Universal screening and treatment strategies in asymptomatic women

Although only about 30% of low-risk women with a short cervix deliver before 35 weeks' gestation, there is evidence that screening all pregnant women for cervical length in the late second trimester and treating women with a short cervix have potential to improve outcome. Vaginal progesterone has been shown to reduce preterm birth in two clinical trials of 'universal' screening [23,24]. In contrast, Grobman et al [25] found that 17 α-hydroxyprogesterone (a synthetic progestagen given by intramuscular injection–– not licensed in the UK) did not reduce the frequency of spontaneous preterm birth in nulliparous women with a cervical length <30 mm.

Cervical length screening in low and mixed populations and treating with cervical cerclage have also been found to be ineffective [26]. These results were confirmed in an individual patient data (IPD) meta-analysis of four trials of cerclage versus expectant management in women with a short cervix [27].

An alternative promising treatment is the cervical pessary (Arabin), which is purported to change the angle of cervix in relation to the uterus, thus reducing pressure on the cervix as well as decreasing contact between fetal membranes and vaginal bacteria, thereby prolonging pregnancy. Goya et al performed a multicentre trial and found that the rate of spontaneous delivery before 34 weeks of gestation was lower in the pessary group than in the expectant management group [7]. No adverse effects were noted, apart from mild discomfort upon insertion, and vaginal discharge.

Despite the positive results relating to cervical length screening and vaginal progesterone or cervical pessary, many unanswered questions remain. At present, universal screening for preterm labour is neither recommended by the UK National Screening Committee or NICE in the UK nor by the American College of Obstetrics and Gynaecology and Society of Maternal and Fetal Medicine in the United States. This is due to concerns over availability of screening, the potential for women to receive unnecessary or unproven interventions and questions over quality assurance. There is an absence of good data comparing screening with no screening and further research is needed including evaluation of cost-effectiveness before universal screening for spontaneous preterm birth should be implemented.

Targeted screening and treatment strategies in asymptomatic women

The predictive performance of a test depends on the characteristics of the population being tested, with higher positive predictive values seen in populations at higher risk. Thus, the positive predictive value of cervical length and fibronectin testing is higher in women at high risk of spontaneous preterm birth.

The clinical risk factor most strongly associated with spontaneous preterm birth is a history of previous preterm delivery, whilst a history of cervical treatment for cervical intraepithelial neoplasia (CIN) (such as large loop excision of the transformation zone) similarly increases the risk of preterm birth [28A]. Specialised clinics for such women have been advocated as a means of improving maternal and neonatal outcomes with protocols for cervical length and/or fFN screening, and prophylactic treatment for women with positive test results. However the benefits of such specialised clinics in achieving these aims remain unproven.

Although there is no clear evidence that specialised antenatal clinics reduce the number of preterm births, they are now accepted as part of care in many settings [28B]. However, the best approach to the management of women at high risk of spontaneous preterm labour remains unclear. This is evidenced in a recent survey of UK practice, which showed wide variation in the provision of specialist services for women at high risk of preterm birth, and heterogeneity in the management of such women [29]. Systematic reviews and IPD meta-analysis have suggested that both cervical cerclage [27] and vaginal progesterone reduce preterm delivery in women with a short cervix who have had a previous preterm delivery [5]. The limited data available comparing treatments in women with a previous preterm birth and a short cervix suggest similar effectiveness of treatments [30]. More research is needed to determine optimal management for women at high risk of preterm labour.

Screening and treatment in women with multiple pregnancies

Although women with multiple pregnancies are at high risk of spontaneous preterm labour, preventative treatments have been largely ineffective at improving outcomes in this group. Cervical cerclage does not reduce preterm birth or improve neonatal outcome in women with multiple pregnancies [31]. Trials of progesterone have also shown no benefit in multiple pregnancies overall, but there is suggestion of a reduction in adverse perinatal outcome seen with progesterone treatment in a subgroup of women with a cervical length ≤25 mm [32]. Furthermore, in a randomised trial of the cervical pessary in women with twins [33], although the pessary did not reduce preterm birth or the primary neonatal composite outcome overall, both were significantly reduced in a prespecified subgroup of women with a cervical length <25th centile. Further research is required to confirm whether progesterone or other treatments such as the cervical pessary would be of benefit in women with multiple pregnancies and a short cervix, and whether strategies of cervical length screening in women with multiple pregnancies may be of benefit.

PREDICTION OF PRETERM LABOUR IN SYMPTOMATIC WOMEN

Cervical length as a predictor of preterm birth in symptomatic women

Despite the relatively promising LRs associated with cervical length measurement for the prediction of preterm birth in women with symptoms suggestive of preterm labour found in the systematic review by Honest et al [12], there is limited evidence of the effectiveness in clinical practice. A Cochrane systematic review of cervical assessment by ultrasound for preventing preterm delivery included three trials of women with singleton gestations and signs and symptoms of preterm labour [34]. Knowledge of cervical length did not have any effect on maternal or neonatal outcomes. The authors concluded that this may relate to the small number of trials, although it may also reflect the lack of effective treatments to prevent preterm delivery in this group.

fFN as a predictor of preterm birth in symptomatic women

A recent systematic review of fFN testing in symptomatic women [14] included analysis of test accuracy, and of the clinical effectiveness and cost-effectiveness of fFN in women with signs and symptoms suggestive of preterm labour. The sensitivity of fFN testing was highest for predicting preterm deliveries within 7–10 days of testing. Estimates of overall sensitivity and specificity for the accuracy of fFN testing to predict preterm delivery within 7–10 days of testing in women with threatened preterm labour were 76.7% (95% CI 70.4–82.0%) and 82.7% (95% CI 79.4–85.5%) respectively. Although only moderate sensitivity was evident in an analysis of the findings of five randomised control trials of fFN (four published trials and one published abstract), no increases in adverse outcomes were found. This may be because fibronectin is only one component included in clinical decision-making, and in most studies, the decision to administer treatment was at the discretion of the clinician. Meta-analysis of the findings of the clinical trials of fFN found no significant differences in incidence of preterm birth, hospital admission or administration of treatment. There was some limited evidence that including fFN in the diagnostic workup may reduce resource use. A recent publication has suggested that quantitative fFN may perform better than qualitative fFN for the prediction of spontaneous preterm birth in women with symptoms suggestive of preterm labour, and help further distinguish women at very low likelihood of delivery [35]. Management guidelines based on this study have been developed by hospitals using the test and examples are available from the manufacturer Hologic (hologic. com). **Table 2.2** shows the St Thomas's Hospital London Preterm Birth Management Protocol. Further research is needed to confirm how to interpret fibronectin concentrations and which thresholds should be used to guide management.

fFN value (ng/ mL)	% who will deliver in 2 weeks	% who will deliver at <34 weeks	Management guidelines 24 + 0 to 34 + 6 weeks
10–49	<2	<2	Discharge with routine midwife follow-up
		5–15	Discharge with routine consultant follow-up
50–199	5–15	10–15	• Admit • Give betamethasone 12 mg IM 12 hours apart
200–499	30	30	• Admit • Give betamethasone 12 mg IM 12 hours apart • Tocolysis with nifedipine 20 mg stat then 10 mg QDS for 24 hours
>500	50	75	• Admit • Give betamethasone 12 mg IM 12 hours apart • Tocolysis with nifedipine 20 mg stat then 10 mg QDS for 24 hours • Magnesium sulphate 4 g IV over 20 minutes and then 1 g/h for 24 hours or until delivery, whichever is sooner

Table 2.2 St Thomas's Hospital, London Spontaneous Preterm Birth Management Protocol

fFN has similar predictive ability both in women with multiple pregnancies and singleton pregnancies [36]. fFN appears to retain its diagnostic performance in patients with a cervical cerclage, and sensitivity and negative predictive values are comparable, although there may be a higher false-positive rate [37].

Sequential cervical length and fFN testing

A systematic review has suggested that combined cervical length screening and qualitative fFN may be a useful strategy for identifying women with symptoms of preterm labour who are unlikely to deliver early [38]. This has been tested in a prospective cohort study of 714 women in the Netherlands [39]. The results indicated that women with a cervical length of <30 mm or with a cervical length between 15 and 30 mm and a negative fibronectin result were at low risk (<5%) of spontaneous delivery within 7 days. Fibronectin testing in women with cervical length between 15 and 30 mm additionally classified 103 women (15% of the cohort) as low risk and 36 women (5% of the cohort) as high risk. In a related health economic analysis [40], the authors suggested that implementing fibronectin testing could result in a cost-saving between €2.8 million and €14.4 million in the Netherlands, a country with about 180,000 deliveries annually. However, it should be noted that in the Netherlands it is routine to perform cervical length measurement in women presenting with symptoms of preterm labour. Cervical length measurement has significant resource requirement (estimated NHS cost £68.16 per test) and lack of out-of-hours provision further limits availability in many NHS hospitals, such that in the UK only a small proportion of units include cervical length measurement in the assessment of women with threatened preterm labour [15B]. The cost-effectiveness of sequential cervical length and fFN testing is thus likely to be different in the UK.

Summary of tests for preterm labour in symptomatic women

In summary, although studies of diagnostic test accuracy suggest that both cervical length and fFN may be useful as part of the diagnostic workup of women with threatened preterm labour, there is, as yet, little evidence that in practice they are clinically or cost-effective. Nevertheless, tests of preterm labour are now integrated in UK clinical practice, where their main value relates to their ability to exclude impending delivery, and thus avoid unnecessary, and potentially harmful, treatment. New strategies such as quantitative fFN and combined or sequential cervical length and fFN testing may improve the targeting of treatments aimed at improving outcome.

Key points for clinical practice

- There are currently no good tests for the prediction of spontaneous preterm labour––cervical length and fFN are moderately useful.
- Universal screening for preterm labour in asymptomatic women with either cervical length ultrasound or fFN is not recommended.
- Screening for preterm labour in women at high risk of preterm birth due to a past history of preterm labour or history of cervical treatment has potential to improve outcomes, but more research is needed to define optimal management strategies.
- In women with symptoms of preterm labour, fFN and cervical length may help avoid unnecessary (and potentially harmful) treatment by identifying women who are not likely to deliver early.
- Quantitative fibronectin and sequential testing strategies may further improve targeting of treatments for preterm labour.

REFERENCES

1. Gravett MG, Rubens CE. A framework for strategic investments in research to reduce the global burden of preterm birth. Am J Obstet Gynecol 2012; 207:368–373.
2. Mangham LJ, Petrou S, Doyle LW, et al. The cost of preterm birth throughout childhood in England and Wales. Pediatrics 2009; 123: e312–327.
3. Norman JE, Morris C, Chalmers J. The effect of changing patterns of obstetric care in Scotland (1980-2004) on rates of preterm birth and its neonatal consequences: perinatal database study. PLoS Med 2009; 6:e1000153.
4. Norman JE, Shennan AH. Prevention of preterm birth––why can't we do any better? Lancet 2013; 381:184–185.
5. Dodd JM, Jones L, Flenady V, et al. Prenatal administration of progesterone for preventing preterm birth in women considered to be at risk of preterm birth. Cochrane Syst Rev 2013; 7:CD004947.
6. Alfirevic Z, Stampalija T, Roberts D, et al. Cervical stitch (cerclage) for preventing preterm birth in singleton pregnancy. Cochrane Syst Rev 2012; 4:CD008991.
7. Goya M, Pratcorona L, Merced C, et al. Cervical pessary in pregnant women with a short cervix (PECEP): an open-label randomised controlled trial. Lancet 2012; 379:1800-1806.
8. Roberts D, Dalziel S. Antenatal corticosteroids for accelerating fetal lung maturation for women at risk of preterm birth. Cochrane Database Syst Rev 2006; (3):CD004454.
9. Doyle LW, Crowther CA, Middleton P, et al. Magnesium sulphate for women at risk of preterm birth for neuroprotection of the fetus. Cochrane Database Syst Rev 2009; 1:CD004661.
10. Marlow N, Bennett C, Draper ES, et al. Paerinatal outcomes for extremely preterm babies in relation to place of birth in England: the EPICure 2 study. Arch Dis Child Fetal Neonatal Ed 2014; 99:F181-188.
11. Haas DM, Caldwell DM, Kirkpatrick P, et al. Tocolytic therapy for preterm delivery: systematic review and network meta-analysis. BMJ 2012; 345:e6226.
12. Honest H, Forbes CA, Duree KH, et al. Screening to prevent spontaneous preterm birth: systematic reviews of accuracy and effectiveness literature with economic modelling. Health Technol Assess 2009; 13:1-627.
13. Crane JM and Hutchens D. Transvaginal sonographic measurement of cervical length to predict preterm birth in asymptomatic women at increased risk: a systematic review. Ultrasound Obstet Gynecol 2008; 31:579-587.
14. Deshpande SN, van Asselt AD, Tomini F, et al. Rapid fetal fibronectin testing to predict preterm birth in women with symptoms of premature labour: a systematic review and cost analysis. Health Technol Assess 2013; 17:1-138.
15A. Domin CM, Smith EJ and Terplan M. Transvaginal ultrasonographic measurement of cervical length as a predictor of preterm birth: a systematic review with meta-analysis. Ultrasound Q 2010: 26:241-248.
15B. Stock SJ, Morris RK, Chandiramani M, et al. Variation in management of women with threatened preterm labour. Arch Dis Child Fetal Neonatal Ed. 2014 Dec 19. [Epub ahead of print].
16. Iams JD, Goldenberg RL, Meis PJ, et al. The length of the cervix and the risk of spontaneous premature delivery. National Institute of Child Health and Human Development Maternal Fetal Medicine Unit Network. N Engl J Med 1996; 334:567-572.
17. Melamed N, Hiersch L, Meizner I, et al. Is cervical length an accurate predictive tool in women with a history of preterm delivery who present with threatened preterm labor? Ultrasound Obstet Gynecol 2014; 44:661–668.
18. Hernandez-Andrade E, Romero R, Ahn H, et al. Transabdominal evaluation of uterine cervical length during pregnancy fails to identify a substantial number of women with a short cervix. J Matern Fetal Neonatal Med 2012; 25:1682-1689.
19. Owen J, Neely C, Northen A. Transperineal versus endovaginal ultrasonographic examination of the cervix in the midtrimester: a blinded comparison. Am J Obstet Gynecol 1999; 181:780–783.
20. Kurtzman J, Chandiramani M, Briley A, et al. Quantitative fetal fibronectin screening in asymptomatic high-risk patients and the spectrum of risk for recurrent preterm delivery. Am J Obstet Gynecol 2009; 200:263. e261-266.
21. Abbott DS, Hezelgrave NL, Seed PT, et al. Quantitative Fetal Fibronectin to Predict Preterm Birth in Asymptomatic Women at High Risk. Obstet Gynecol 2015; doi: 10.1097/AOG.0000000000000754.
22. Abbott DH, Seed NL, Bennett PT, et al. EQUIPP: Evaluation of Fetal Fibronectin with a novel bedside Quantitative Instrument for the Prediction of Preterm birth. Arch Dis Child Fetal Neonatal Ed 2014; 99:A150–A151.

23. Fonseca EB, Celik E, Parra M, et al. Progesterone and the risk of preterm birth among women with a short cervix. N Engl J Med 2007; 357:462-469.
24. Hassan SS, Romero R, Vidyadhari D, et al. Vaginal progesterone reduces the rate of preterm birth in women with a sonographic short cervix: a multicenter, randomized, double-blind, placebo-controlled trial. Ultrasound Obstet Gynecol 2011; 38:18-31.
25. Grobman WA, Thom EA, Spong CY, et al. 17 alpha-hydroxyprogesterone caproate to prevent prematurity in nulliparas with cervical length less than 30 mm. Am J Obstet Gynecol 2012; 207:390 e391-398.
26. To MS, Alfirevic Z, Heath VC, et al. Cervical cerclage for prevention of preterm delivery in women with short cervix: randomised controlled trial. Lancet 2004; 363:1849-1853.
27. Berghella V, Roman A, Daskalakis C, et al. Gestational age at cervical length measurement and incidence of preterm birth. Obstet Gynecol 2007; 110:311-317.
28A.Stock S, Norman J. Treatments for precursors of cervical cancer and preterm labour. BJOG 2012;119:647–649.
28B.Whitworth M, Quenby S, Cockerill RO, et al. Specialised antenatal clinics for women with a pregnancy at high risk of preterm birth (excluding multiple pregnancy) to improve maternal and infant outcomes. Cochrane Syst Rev 2011; 9:CD006760.
29. Sharp AN and Alfirevic Z. Provision and practice of specialist preterm labour clinics: a UK survey of practice. BJOG 2014; 121:417-421.
30. Alfirevic Z, Owen J, Carreras Moratonas E, et al. Vaginal progesterone, cerclage or cervical pessary for preventing preterm birth in asymptomatic singleton pregnant women with a history of preterm birth and a sonographic short cervix. Ultrasound Obstet Gynecol 2013; 41:146-151.
31. Rafael TJ, Berghella V, Alfirevic Z. Cervical stitch (cerclage) for preventing preterm birth in multiple pregnancy. Cochrane Database Syst Rev 2014; 9:CD009166.
32. Schuit E, Stock S, Rode L, et al. Effectiveness of progestogens to improve perinatal outcome in twin pregnancies: an individual participant data meta-analysis. BJOG 2015; 122:27–37.
33. Liem S, Schuit E, Hegeman M, et al. Cervical pessaries for prevention of preterm birth in women with a multiple pregnancy (ProTWIN): a multicentre, open-label randomised controlled trial. Lancet 2013; 382:1341-1349.
34. Berghella V, Baxter JK, Hendrix NW. Cervical assessment by ultrasound for preventing preterm delivery. Cochrane Database Syst Rev 2013; 1:CD007235.
35. Abbott DS, Radford SK, Seed PT, et al. Evaluation of a quantitative fetal fibronectin test for spontaneous preterm birth in symptomatic women. Am J Obstet Gynecol 2013; 208:122 e121-126.
36. Singer E, Pilpel S, Bsat F, et al. Accuracy of fetal fibronectin to predict preterm birth in twin gestations with symptoms of labor. Obstet Gynecol 2007; 109:1083-1087.
37. Duhig KE, Chandiramani M, Seed PT, et al. Fetal fibronectin as a predictor of spontaneous preterm labour in asymptomatic women with a cervical cerclage. BJOG 2009; 116:799-803.
38. DeFranco EA, Lewis DF and Odibo AO. Improving the screening accuracy for preterm labor: is the combination of fetal fibronectin and cervical length in symptomatic patients a useful predictor of preterm birth? A systematic review. Am J of Obstet Gynecol 2013; 208:233 e231-236.
39. van Baaren GJ, Vis JY, Wilms FF, et al. Predictive value of cervical length measurement and fibronectin testing in threatened preterm labor. Obstet Gynecol 2014; 123:1185-1192.
40. van Baaren GJ, Vis JY, Grobman WA, et al. Cost-effectiveness analysis of cervical length measurement and fibronectin testing in women with threatened preterm labor. Am J Obstet Gynecol 2013; 209: 36 e431-438.

Chapter 3

Medical management of endometriosis

Arne Vanhie, Carla Tomassetti, Christel Meuleman, Thomas D'Hooghe

INTRODUCTION

Women with endometriosis are confronted with one or both of two major problems: endometriosis-associated pain and infertility [1]. Although endometriosis is a benign gynaecological disorder, its treatment is complex and often frustrating due to the progressive character and high recurrence rates of endometriosis. Management of endometriosis has been based partially on evidence-based practices and partially on unsubstantiated therapies and approaches. Guidelines have been developed by a number of national and international bodies, yet areas of controversy and uncertainty remain, not at least due to a paucity of firm evidence [2A].

In 2008, the Practice Committee of the American Society of Reproductive Medicine (ASRM) stated that 'endometriosis should be viewed as a chronic disease that requires a life-long management with the goal of maximizing the use of medical treatment and avoiding repeated surgical procedures' [2B,35]. In this chapter, we will provide an overview of the medical management of endometriosis. We will review the use of medical therapies in the management of endometriosis-associated pain and prevention of endometriosis, with the emphasis on evidence-based practice. In the final section, an overview of novel agents and future directions of medical treatment of endometriosis is presented.

Endometriosis originates from retrograde menstruation of endometrial tissue sloughed through patent fallopian tubes into the peritoneal cavity [3]. These steroid-hormone sensitive endometrial cells and tissues implant on the peritoneal surface and elicit an inflammatory response [3]. This response is accompanied by angiogenesis, adhesions, fibrosis, scarring, neuronal infiltration and anatomical distortion, resulting in pain and infertility [3]. This process of retrograde menstruation, peritoneal implantation and chronic inflammation is presumed to occur against a predisposing background of genetic, environmental and immunological factors, since most women have some degree of retrograde menstruation, but only 6–10% have endometriosis [3]. It is hypothesised that

Arne Vanhie MD, Department of Obstetrics and Gynaecology, University Hospital Leuven, Leuven, Belgium

Carla Tomassetti MD, Department of Obstetrics and Gynaecology, University Hospital Leuven, Leuven, Belgium

Christel Meuleman MD PhD, Department of Obstetrics and Gynaecology, University Hospital Leuven, Leuven, Belgium

Thomas D'Hooghe MD PhD, Department of Obstetrics and Gynaecology, University Hospital Leuven, Leuven, Belgium. Email: thomas.dhooghe@uzleuven.be (for correspondence)

the endometrium of women with endometriosis is predisposed to successful establishment of ectopic disease and that the immune system in women with endometriosis is altered, resulting in a reduced immunological clearance of viable endometrial cells from the pelvic cavity [4A,4B]. Although the underlying etiological mechanism remains uncertain, these important insights into the pathophysiology of endometriosis have led to the recognition of possible new targets for medical therapies.

Medical treatment of endometriosis should ideally eradicate endometriosis rather than merely relieving its symptoms [35]. However, in the light of the transplantation theory, it seems very difficult to develop a cytoreductive compound which can effectively eliminate endometriotic lesions without carrying a high risk of damage to the eutopic endometrium [35]. Currently available medications result in suppression of endometriosis rather than cytoreduction and attempt to achieve main objectives: relief of symptoms (pain) for prolonged periods and prevention of disease progression [35].

MEDICAL THERAPIES IN THE MANAGEMENT OF ENDOMETRIOSIS-ASSOCIATED PAIN

Pharmacodynamics

The paramount role of oestrogens in the maintenance of endometriosis is demonstrated by several clinical observations and concurs with the transplantation theory of oestrogen-dependent eutopic endometrium [4C]. First, epidemiological data show that endometriosis predominantly affects women during the reproductive phase of life and that endometriosis regresses after menopause support the oestrogen-dependence hypothesis [4C]. Furthermore, the administration of hormone replacement therapy may cause relapse of the disease in some postmenopausal women [4C]. In premenopausal women, the suppression of oestradiol secretion by administration of gonadotropin-releasing hormone analogues (GnRH-a) causes regression of endometriotic lesions and improvement of pain symptoms [4C]. Moreover, the recovery of oestradiol secretion after discontinuation of the therapy is associated with relapse of the disease, underscoring the oestrogen-dependent character of endometriosis [4C].

The clinical observation of apparent symptom resolution during pregnancy gave rise to the concept of treating patients with a pseudopregnancy regime [5A]. In 1958, Kistner was the first to use combinations of high-dose oestrogens and progestogens, and later progestogens alone [5A]. Nowadays, high doses of oestrogen and progesterone are rarely prescribed and modern low-dose preparations are widely used in the treatment of endometriosis. Decidualisation followed by atrophy of both the eutopic and ectopic endometrial tissue is the generic proposed mechanism of action [5B]. Additionally, combined oral contraceptives (COCs) might have a positive effect on endometriosis through reduction of menstrual blood flow and downregulation of cell proliferation and enhancement of programmed cell death in the eutopic endometrium [6].

Similar to COCs, the chronic administration of progestins results in decidualisation and subsequent atrophy of endometrial tissue [5B]. Recent research also suggests a possible role of progestogen-induced suppression of matrix metalloproteinases, a class of enzymes important in the growth and implantation of ectopic endometrium, and inhibition of angiogenesis [5B].

GnRH agonists are synthetic analogues of GnRH that differ from the native hormone with respect to the specific amino acid sequence [7]. All are designed to either increase receptor affinity or decrease GnRH degradation [7]. Their use therefore leads to persistent activation of GnRH receptors [7]. This activation results in an initial release of gonadotropins previously produced and stored in the pituitary [7]. However, the release is rapidly followed by downregulation of GnRH receptor expression and profound suppression of gonadotropin secretion [7]. As a result, sex-steroid production in the ovary falls to levels similar to those seen after castration [7]. This profound hypoestrogenic state inhibits the development, maintenance and growth of endometriosis, which in turn alters the effect on the immune, nervous and endocrine systems. The hypoestrogenemia also has direct effects on these systems, further altering their status from that seen in patients with active endometriosis [7].

The hypoestrogenism induced by GnRH agonists can result in bone loss and severe hypoestrogenic symptoms [1]. To reduce the negative effects of oestrogen deprivation, hormonal add-back therapy with oestrogens and/or progestogens or tibolone is recommended [1]. This is based on the threshold theory, by which lower oestrogen levels are needed to protect the bone and cognitive function and to avoid/minimise menopausal symptoms than to activate endometriotic tissue [8].

Aromatase inhibitors (AIs) constitute another class of drugs that cause hypoestrogenism and are used in the treatment of endometriosis. AIs suppress oestradiol production through reversible (anastrozole, letrozole) or irreversible (exemestane) inhibition of the aromatase P450 enzyme resulting in hypoestrogenism [4B]. The enzyme aromatase P450 plays an important role in the production of oestradiol where it converts androstenedione to oestrone (E1) (reviewed by Ferrerro [4C]). Subsequently, E1 is converted to oestradiol (E2) by the activity of 17-OH-steroid dehydrogenase (reviewed by Ferrerro [4C]). E2 is mainly produced by the ovary in a cyclic fashion, where it is secreted by the preovulatory follicle. In addition, in peripheral tissues (such as fat, skin and skeletal muscle), there is conversion of circulating androstenedione of adrenal origin to E1 (reviewed by Ferrerro [4C]). Endometriotic tissue, unlike disease-free endometrium, exhibits a high level of aromatase activity that may result in increased local concentrations of oestradiol that may favour the growth of endometriosis [5,9].

Evidence and recommendations

Women suffering from chronic pelvic pain, dysmenorrhoea and dyspareunia with a high suspicion of endometriosis are often prescribed hormonal medication and analgesics without a prior definitive laparoscopic diagnosis [1]. It is common practice for laparoscopy to be performed if the patient does not react favourably to the prescribed medical or hormonal treatment. However in a retrospective study, relief of chronic pelvic pain symptoms, or lack of response, with preoperative hormonal therapy was not an accurate predictor of the presence or absence of histologically confirmed endometriosis at laparoscopy [10]. Furthermore, empirical treatment can lead to a delay in diagnosis associated with significant social and psychological disadvantages [10]. Notwithstanding the drawbacks to use of empirical treatment rather than early use of laparoscopy, laparoscopy carries small but significant surgical and anaesthetic risk. The ESHRE 2013 guideline still considers empirical treatment as good clinical practice provided that the patient has been counselled thoroughly about the possibility of endometriosis and that other causes of pelvic pain have been ruled out as thoroughly as possible [1].

The first-line medical treatment for pain due to endometriosis is often a nonsteroidal anti-inflammatory drug (NSAID). Good evidence exists to support the use of NSAIDs for primary dysmenorrhoea, [11], but a Cochrane meta-analysis from 2009 concluded that there are insufficient data to show that NSAIDs significantly reduce endometriosis pain [12]. It has to be noted that only two studies were available that investigated the role of NSAIDs in the relief of endometriosis-associated pain [12]. Nevertheless, the ESHRE 2013 guideline recommends that clinicians should consider NSAIDs or other analgesics to reduce endometriosis-associated pain, due to the known benefit of NSAIDs in primary dysmenorrhoea. [1].

There is strong evidence that suppression of ovarian function reduces pain associated with endometriosis. Currently COCs, progestogens, antiprogestogens, GnRH agonists and AIs are in clinical use [1]. There is no evidence to support the superiority of one product to the other, but side effects and cost profiles differ [35]. Hence, it is recommended that clinicians take patient preferences, side effects, costs and availability into consideration when choosing hormonal treatment for endometriosis-associated pain.

A Cochrane systematic review from 2007 addressed the use of COCs for pain associated with endometriosis [13]. Surprisingly, only one study was found and included, despite the widespread use of COC in clinical practice [14]. In the included study, no significant difference between treatment with COC and GnRH agonist was seen [14]. Based on this study and on the widespread use of COCs, both the 2013 ESHRE and the [5B] guideline recommend the consideration of a COC, vaginal contraceptive ring or transdermal patch in the treatment of endometriosis-associated pain.

The body of evidence supporting the use of progestogens and antiprogestogens in the treatment of endometriosis-associated pain is larger than for COCs. In their systematic review from 2012, Brown et al included 13 papers evaluating progestogens and antiprogestogens [15]. Of the two studies comparing progestogens with placebo, only one showed a significant effect. There was no overall evidence of a benefit of progestogens over other medical treatments (COCs, GnRH agonists). Amenorrhoea and bleeding were more frequently reported in the progestogen group compared with other treatment groups. The authors conclude that the evidence for progestogens in the treatment of endometriosis pain is limited [15]. The 2013 ESHRE guideline considered this evidence as sufficient to recommend the use of progestogens (medroxyprogesterone acetate, dienogest, cyproterone acetate, norethisterone acetate, levonorgestrel-releasing intrauterine system or danazol) and antiprogestogens (gestrinone) [1]. However, the guidelines stress that clinicians should take the side effects of progestogens and antiprogestogens into account when prescribing these drugs [1]. Due to its severe side effects (acne, oedema, vaginal spotting, weight gain, muscle cramps), the use of danazol is discouraged, and should only be considered if no other medical therapy is available [1].

GnRH agonists have been studied more extensively for the treatment of endometriosis-associated pain than other medical therapies [7]. Multiple randomised trials have compared GnRH agonists with other treatments for endometriosis, including COCs, progestogens and danazol. A Cochrane review compared GnRH agonists at different doses, regimens and routes of administration, with danazol, intrauterine progestogen, placebo and analgesics for relieving endometriosis-associated pain symptoms [16]. According to this review, GnRH agonists were superior to placebo, but inferior to the levonorgestrel-releasing intrauterine system or danazol. Also the review indicated a worse side-effect profile for GnRH agonists, mainly menopausal symptoms related to severe hypoestrogenemia (bone loss, hot flushes, vaginal dryness) and no difference according to route of administration of the GnRH agonist [16]. Several studies have explored whether add-back therapy reduces the side effects of GnRH agonist treatment, although large randomised controlled trials (RCTs) are absent [17A-20]. These studies suggest a reduction in side effects by adding oestrogens and/or progestogens and none of these trials reported a negative effect of add-back therapy on the efficacy of treatment with GnRH agonists [17A-20]. It can be concluded that GnRH agonists, with and without add-back therapy, are effective in the relief of endometriosis-associated pain, but evidence is limited regarding dosage or duration of treatment and severe side effects should be taken into account when prescribing these drugs without add-back therapy [1].

Even though the evidence for increased expression of aromatase P450 in endometriotic tissue is still controversial, AIs have been studied as treatment for pain symptoms in premenopausal women with endometriosis [1]. A systematic review evaluating the use of AIs to treat endometriosis-associated pain concluded that the existing evidence is of moderate quality and that evidence on the long-term effects is lacking [21]. Like GnRH agonists without add-back, AIs have severe side effects such as vaginal dryness, hot flushes and diminished bone density. Furthermore, in premenopausal women, AIs lead to an increase in follicle-stimulating hormone levels and subsequent follicular development and therefore must be used in combination with other agents (progestogens, COCs or GnRH agonists) to downregulate the ovaries [5B]. Treatment of endometriosis-associated pain with AIs should be considered investigational and only be prescribed to women after all other options for medical or surgical treatment are exhausted [1,5].

MEDICAL THERAPIES IN THE PREVENTION OF ENDOMETRIOSIS

Primary prevention

Primary prevention is defined as those measures that protect healthy individuals from developing the disease. A typical example is immunisation against infectious diseases, but it also includes health promotion and regulation of environmental pollutants (Novak's Gynaecology, Minerva EBM).

Given that the exact cause and pathogenesis of endometriosis are unknown, potential interventions for primary prevention are limited [1]. In light of the retrograde menstruation theory, the use of COCs for primary prevention has been suggested [36]. COCs suppress ovulation and substantially reduce the amount of monthly uterine blood flow. They are successfully used in the treatment of pain symptoms, and progestogens may inhibit expression of matrix metalloproteinases and angiogenesis. The relationship between COC use and risk of endometriosis was evaluated in a systematic review by Vercellini et al in 2011 [36]. The authors conclude that the risk of endometriosis appears reduced during OC use, but that it is not possible to exclude the possibility that the apparent protective effect of COC against endometriosis is the result of postponement of surgical evaluation due to temporary suppression of pain symptoms [36]. Based on this meta-analysis, the ESHRE guidelines state that the usefulness of OCs for the primary prevention of endometriosis is uncertain [1].

A second factor that has been investigated is the possible link between the level of physical activity and endometriosis [1]. Physical activity has been hypothesised to be protective against endometriosis because it may increase levels of sex hormone binding globulin, which would reduce bioavailable oestrogens, and it reduces insulin resistance and hyperinsulinemia, which has been hypothesised to be related to endometriosis [22]. Several case–control studies reported a strong risk reduction of endometriosis associated with physical activity [23-26]. However a study based on prospective collected data from the Nurses' Health Study II [22] did not replicate these strong associations. They observed a weak protective effect among fertile participants for total recreational physical activity reported 2 years before diagnosis and a slightly stronger protective effect for aerobic exercise on the rate of laparoscopically confirmed endometriosis [22]. Based on these prospective data, the ESHRE guideline states that the usefulness of physical exercise for the primary prevention of endometriosis is uncertain [1].

Secondary prevention

Secondary preventive measures are those interventions that are used to diagnose the disease in an early (preclinical) stage or when the diagnosis has been established to prevent recurrences, exacerbations or complications of the disease and its treatment. Examples of secondary preventive measures are well known in gynaecology such as screening mammography and cervical cytology testing (Novak Gynaecology). In the ESHRE guideline, secondary prevention of endometriosis was defined as prevention of the recurrence of pain symptoms (dysmenorrhoea, dyspareunia, nonmenstrual pelvic pain) or the recurrence of disease (recurrence of endometriosis lesions documented by ultrasound for ovarian endometrioma or by laparoscopy for all endometriosis lesions) in the long term (>6 months after surgery) [1].

A frustrating aspect of surgical treatment of endometriosis is the variable recurrence rate of between 10% and 55% within 12 months after excision/removal by an expert in endometriosis surgery, with an extra 10% of recurrence for each additional year after surgery [2A]. Hence there has been considerable interest in the effectiveness of pre- and postoperative medical therapies for lowering recurrence and complication rates after surgical treatment of endometriosis. However, as discussed earlier, currently available medical treatment does not eradicate but suppress endometriosis, and often there is a relapse after discontinuation of treatment [27]. Therefore, adjuvant therapies for secondary prevention need to be administered for a long-time course and should be safe, well tolerated and relatively inexpensive. OCs and progestogens may be the best pharmacological options [35].

Several studies have investigated the value of pre- and postoperative medical therapy. A Cochrane review considered both pre- and postoperative treatment in relation to the management of cysts, pain and infertility. The authors conclude that there was no evidence of a benefit of preoperative medical therapy on the outcome of surgery [28]. The ESHRE guideline endorses that preoperative treatment with GnRH-a to facilitate surgery is common clinical practice, although there are no controlled studies supporting this [1]. Based on the same Cochrane review, both the ESHRE and ASRM guidelines recommend the use of postoperative hormonal treatment (COC, levonorgestrel-releasing intra-uterine device, progestogens) for the secondary prevention of recurrence of both symptoms and lesions [1,5]. It is important to note that postoperative medical treatment does not improve outcome of surgery and as such there is no clear rationale for short-term (<6 months) adjuvant treatment after surgery [1].

NOVEL AGENTS AND FUTURE DIRECTIONS FOR THE MEDICAL TREATMENT OF ENDOMETRIOSIS

Novel targets for hormonal treatment

Selective oestrogen receptor modulators (SERMs) are chemically diverse compounds that lack the steroid structure of oestrogens but possess a tertiary structure that allows them to bind to the oestrogen receptor. Unlike oestrogens, which are uniformly agonists, and antioestrogens, which are uniformly antagonists, the SERMs exert selective agonist or antagonist effects on various oestrogen target tissues [29]. The role of SERMs in the treatment of endometriosis is unclear. In animal models, raloxifene therapy resulted in regression of endometriosis (Novak's Gynaecology). In humans, SERMs have not yet been successful in the treatment of endometriosis. An RCT including women with biopsy-proven endometriosis and chronic pelvic pain treated with raloxifene or placebo was terminated prematurely because the raloxifene group experienced greater pain and had secondary surgery sooner than the placebo group [30]. Another SERM, bazedoxifene, was successful in the treatment of endometriosis in a murine model, but has not been tested in humans (reviewed by Platteeuw [31]).

The large family of progesterone receptor ligands includes pure agonists such as progesterone itself or progestogens and, at the other end of the biological spectrum, pure progesterone receptor antagonists. Selective progesterone receptor modulators (SPRMs) have mixed agonist–antagonist properties, and occupy an intermediate position of the spectrum [32]. Onapristone is a complete antagonist, whereas mifepristone and asoprisnil have mixed effects. Ulipristal acetate has an antagonistic effect on the uterus (reviewed by Platteeuw [31]). SPRMs cause a selective inhibition of endometrial proliferation without oestrogen deprivation and its known side effects (reviewed by Platteeuw [31]). When compared with placebo, treatment of induced endometriosis in rats with onapristone or ulipristal acetate reduced both volume and weight of lesions (<50%), comparable with the effect of dienogest or GnRH-a (reviewed by Platteeuw [31]). In monkeys, surgically induced endometriotic lesions were reduced after 9 months of mifepristone treatment [32]. Three small clinical trials have been reported using mifepristone in humans [32]. There was an improvement in symptoms in all treated patients independently of the dose and a 55% mean regression of visible endometriosis after 6 months of treatment with 50 mg/day [32]. Given that asoprisnil and onapristone were withdrawn because of endometrial side effects and/or severe hepatic toxicity, the potential value of mifepristone, telapristone and ulipristal acetate remains to be established with respect to safety and efficacy in the treatment of endometriosis in humans (reviewed by Platteeuw [31]).

Novel targets for nonhormonal treatment

The importance of chronic inflammation, angiogenesis and immunological changes in the pathophysiology of endometriosis has been discussed earlier. Although the exact underlying mechanisms are unclear, medical therapies targeting these different pathways are being investigated. Most of this research has been done in rodent models with induced endometriosis. Therefore, the safety and efficacy remain to be established in studies performed in relevant and standardised preclinical models such as the baboon model [33,34].

A first group of drugs currently under investigation are anti-inflammatory agents targeting endometriosis-associated peritoneal inflammation. Inhibition of COX-2 synthesis can reduce PGE-2 synthesis and oestrogen production. Selective inhibitors of COX-2 have the property to block the growth of ectopic cells and induce apoptosis. Due to severe side effects, rofecoxib and valdecoxib have been withdrawn from the market. Other COX-2 inhibitors have been tested for endometriosis treatment in mice but not in humans. Antioxidants have been tested in small, nonrandomised clinical trials showing small effects, but large RCTs with sufficient power are needed to further evaluate their role. Metformin and thiazolidinediones are widely used antidiabetic drugs with, next to their insulin-sensitizing effects, anti-inflammatory properties and have been effective in treating endometriosis in rat models (reviewed by Platteeuw [31]).

Another possible therapeutic strategy is the inhibition of cytokines with specific antibodies. In mice with induced endometriosis, administration of a macrophage migrating inhibitory factor antagonist led to a significant decline of the number, size and in situ dissemination of endometriotic lesions compared with placebo. Antitumor necrosis factor alpha was effective in baboons, but its effect remains to be studied in humans, as a small RCT did not show a benefit for pelvic pain in women awaiting surgery for deep endometriosis (reviewed by Platteeuw [31]).

Antiangiogenesis agents targeting the neovascularisation of endometriotic lesions including statins, antivascular endothelial growth factor, curcumin, dopamine receptor antagonists and gene therapy have all been evaluated (reviewed by Platteeuw [31]). Statins in high doses have been shown to exhibit antiangiogenic activity and were effective for treatment of endometriosis in mouse models. Treatment of rats with induced endometriosis with a monoclonal antibody against VEGF, the most important angiogenic factor involved in the pathogenesis of endometriosis, resulted in decreased volume of endometriotic implants (reviewed by Platteeuw [31]).

The activation of nuclear factor (NF)-κB and proteasome pathways participates in the pathophysiology of endometriosis by inducing growth and inflammation of endometriotic lesions. Pyrrolidine dithiocarbamate (PDTC) is an antioxidant and potent NF-κB inhibitor. Treatment of rats with induced endometriosis with PDTC reduced endometriotic lesion volume significantly in comparison to placebo treatment (reviewed by Platteeuw [31]).

Many other substances potentially capable of modulating immunological or inflammatory mechanisms involved in the onset or progression of endometriosis could be the targets for future research. As for the drugs discussed in the last paragraphs, the efficacy and safety of these possible new therapies needs to be thoroughly evaluated in animal models and humans. Furthermore, these novel agents must be shown to be safe for long-term use, as endometriosis is a chronic disease requiring long-term therapy.

Key points for clinical practice

- Current medical therapies of endometriosis are based on its oestrogen dependent character. Hypoestrogenism leads to decidualisation and atrophy of endometriotic lesions.
- There is strong evidence that suppression of ovarian function reduces pain associated with endometriosis.
- Currently COCs, progestogens, antiprogestogens, GnRH agonists and AIs are in clinical use. There is no evidence to support the superiority of one product to the other, but side effects and cost profiles differ.

- When using GnRH-agonists, hormonal add-back therapy should be prescribed to prevent bone loss and hypoestrogenic symptoms.
- At present there is no sufficient evidence to support the use of oral contraceptives for primary prevention of endometriosis.
- Post-operative hormonal treatment is recommended for prevention of recurrence after surgery for endometriosis (secondary prevention).

REFERENCES

1. Dunselman GA, Vermeulen N, Becker C, et al. ESHRE Guidelines: management of women with endometriosis. Hum Reprod 2014;29:400–412.
2A. Johnson N, Hummolshoj L. Consensus on current management of endometriosis. Hum Reprod 2013;28:1552–1568.
2B. Practice Committee of American Society for Reproductive Medicine. Treatment of pelvic pain associated with endometriosis. Fertil Setril 2008; 90:S260-269.
3. Giudice L. Endometriosis. N Engl J Med 2010;362:2389–2398.
4A. Giudice LC and Kao LC. Endometriosis. Lancet 2004; 13-9,364:1789-1799.
4B. Burney RO and Giudice LC. Pathogenesis and pathophysiology of endometriosis. Fertil Steril 2012; 98:511-519.
4C. Ferrero S, Remorgida V, Maganza C, et al. Aromatase and endometriosis: estrogens play a role. Ann N Y Acad Sci 2014; 1317:17–23.
5A. Davis L, Kennedy SS, Moore J, et al. Modern combined oral contraceptives for pain associated with endometriosis. Cochrane Database Syst Rev 2007; 18:CD001019.
5B. ASRM Practice Committee. Treatment of pelvic pain associated with endometriosis: a committee opinion. Fertil Steril 2014;101:927–935.
6. Meresman GF, Auge L, Baranao R, et al. Oral contraceptives suppress cell proliferation and enhance apoptosis of eutopic endometrial tissue from patients with endometriosis. Fertil Steril 2002;77:1141–1147.
7. Olive DL. Gonadotropin-releasing hormone agonists for endometriosis. N Engl J Med 2008;359:1136–1142.
8. Barbieri RL. Hormone treatment of endometriosis: the oestrogen threshold hypothesis. AJOG 1992;166:740–745.
9. Bulun SE, Fang Z, Imir G, et al. Aromatase and endometriosis. Semin Reprod Med 2004;22:45–50.
10. Jenkins TR, Liu CY, White J. Does response to hormonal therapy predict presence or absence of endometriosis? J Minim Invasive Gynecol 2008;15:82–86.
11. Marjoribanks J, Proctor M, Farquhar C, et al. Nonsteroidal anti-inflammatory drugs for dysmenorrhoea. Cochrane Database Syst Rev 2010:CD001751.
12. Allen C, Hopewell S, Prentice A, et al. Nonsteroidal anti-inflammatory drugs for pain in women with endometriosis. Cochrane Database Syst Rev 2009:CD004753.
13. Davis L, Kennedy SS, Moore J, et al. Modern combined oral contraceptives for pain associated with endometriosis. Cochrane Database Syst Rev 2007:CD001019.
14. Vercellini P, Trespidi L, Colombo A, et al. A gonadotrophin-releasing hormone agonist versus a low-dose oral contraceptive for pelvic pain associated with endometriosis. Fertil Steril 1993;60:75–79.
15. Brown J, Kives S, Akhtar M. Progestagens and anti-progestagens for pain associated with endometriosis. Cochrane Database Syst Rev 2012;3:CD002122.
16. Brown J, Pan A, Hart RJ. Gonadotrophin-releasing hormone analogues for pain associated with endometriosis. Cochrane Database Syst Rev 2010:CD008475.
17A.Bergqvist A, Jacobson J, Harris S. A double-blind randomized study of the treatment of endometriosis with nafarelin or nafarelin plus norethisterone. Gynecol Endocrinol 1997;11:187–194.
17B.Al-Azemi M, Jones G, Sirkeci F, et al. Immediate and delayed add-back hormonal replacement therapy during ultra long GnRH agonist treatment of chronic pelvic pain. BJOG 2009; 116(12):1646-56.
18. Mäkäräinen L, Rönnberg L, Kauppila A. Medroxyprogesterone acetate supplementation diminishes the hypoestrogenic side effects of gonadotropin-releasing hormone agonist without changing its efficacy in endometriosis. Fertil Steril 1996;65:29–34.

19. Moghissi KS, Schlaff WD, Olive DL, et al. Goserelin acetate (zoladex) with or without hormone replacement therapy for the treatment of endometriosis. Fertil Steril 1998;69:1056–1062.
20. Taskin O, Yalcinoglu AI, Kucuk S, et al. Effectiveness of tibolone on hypoestrogenic symptoms induced by goserelin treatment in patients with endometriosis. Fertil Steril 1997;67:40–45.
21. Ferrero S, Gillott DJ, Venturini PL, et al. Use of aromatase inhibitors to treat endometriosis related pain symptoms: a systematic review. Reprod Biol Endocrinol 2011;9:89–99.
22. Vitonis AF, Hankinson SE, Hornstein MD, et al. Adult physical activity and endometriosis risk. Epidemiology 2010;21:16–23.
23. Cramer DW, Wilson E, Stillman RJ, et al. The relation of endometriosis to menstrual characteristics, smoking, and exercise. JAMA 1986;255:1904–1908.
24. Signorello LB, Harlow BL, Cramer DW, et al. Epidemiologic determinants of endometriosis: a hospital-based case control study. Ann Epidemiol 1997;7:267–741.
25. Dhillon PK, Holt VL. Recreational physical activity and endometrioma risk. Am J Epidemiol 2003;158:156–164.
26. Heilier JF, Donnez J, Nackers F, et al. Environmental and host-associated risk factors in endometriosis and deep endometriotic nodules: a matched case-control study. Environ Res. 2007;103:121–129.
27. Seracchioli R, Mabrouk M, Manuzzi L, et al. Post-operative use of oral contraceptive pills for prevention of anatomical relapse or symptom-recurrence after conservative surgery for endometriosis. Hum Reprod 2009;24:2729–2735.
28. Furness S, Yap C, Farquhar C, et al. Pre and post-operative medical therapy for endometriosis surgery. Cochrane Database Syst Rev 2004:CD003678.
29. Rigg L, Hartmann L. Selective estrogen-receptor modulators: mechanisms of action and application to clinical practice. N Engl J Med 2003;348:618–629.
30. Stratton P, Sinaii N, Segars J, et al. Return of chronic pelvic pain from endometriosis after raloxifene treatment: a randomized controlled trial. Obstet Gynecol 2008;111:88–96.
31. Platteeuw L, D'Hooghe T. Novel agents for the medical treatment of endometriosis. Curr Opin Obstet Gynecol 2014;26:243–252.
32. Chabbert-Buffet N, Meduri G, Bouchard Ph, et al. Selective progesterone receptor modulators and progesterone antagonists: mechanisms of action and clinical applications. Hum Reprod Update 2005;11:293–307.
33. D'Hooghe TM, Debrock S, Kyama CM, et al. Baboon model for fundamental and preclinical research in endometriosis. Gynecol Obstet Invest. 2004;57:43–46.
34. D'Hooghe TM, Kyama CM, Chai D, et al. Nonhuman primate models for translational research in endometriosis. Reprod Sci 2009;16:152–161.
35. Vercellini P, Crosignani PG, Somigliana E, et al. 'Waiting for Godot': a commonsense approach to the medical treatment of endometriosis. Hum Reprod 2011;26:3–13.
36. Vercellini P, Eskenazi B, Consonni D, et al. Oral contraceptives and risk of endometriosis: a systematic review and meta-analysis. Hum Reprod Update 2011;17:159–170.

Chapter 4

Current state of antibody-based immunotherapy for ovarian cancer

*André Fedier, Brian WC Tse, Rosanna Zanetti Dällenbach,
Viola A Heinzelmann-Schwarz*

SUMMARY

Ovarian cancer remains the gynaecological cancer with the highest mortality rate, despite
improvement in outcomes with cytoreductive surgery and platinum-based chemotherapy.
New chemotherapy drugs and particularly the alteration of the delivery cycles have
increased the time over which this disease is controllable. However, novel therapies that
can be integrated into existing treatment regimens are urgently needed. Immunotherapy
is an alternative and rational therapeutic approach for ovarian cancer, based on evidence
supporting a protective role of the immune system and on the clinical success of
immunotherapy in other malignancies. Whether immunotherapy will have a significant
role in the future management of ovarian cancer remains to be seen, but research in this
field is active. In this chapter, the recent clinical developments of selected ovarian cancer-
related immunotherapies fulfilling the criteria that they (1) are antibody based, (2) target a
distinct immunological pathway and (3) have reached the clinical trial stage are discussed
(**Table 4.1**). A particular focus is on catumaxomab (anti-EpCAM x anti-CD3), abagovomab
and oregovomab (anti-CA125), daclizumab (anti-CD25), ipilimumab (anti-CTLA-4), MXD-
1105 (anti-PD-L1) and CVac (anti-mucin1). We will also provide our perspective on the
future of immunotherapy for ovarian cancer and discuss how such immunotherapies may
be best employed in treatment regimens. In addition, recent research will be demonstrated
in an immunotherapy-related field on naturally occurring antiglycan antibodies which
might exhibit further therapeutical opportunities and potential.

André Fedier PhD, Department of Biomedicine, University Hospital Basel, Basel, Switzerland

Brian WC Tse PhD, Australian Prostate Cancer Research Centre-Queensland, Queensland University of Technology, Brisbane, Australia

Rosanna Zanetti Dällenbach PhD, Gynaecological Cancer Center, Women's University Hospital, Basel, Switzerland

Viola A Heinzelmann-Schwarz MD, Department of Biomedicine, University Hospital Basel, Basel, Switzerland; Lowy Cancer Research Centre, University of New South Wales, Sydney, Australia; and Gynaecological Cancer Center, Women's University Hospital, Basel, Switzerland. Email: viola.heinzelmann@usb.ch (for correspondence)

INTRODUCTION

Epithelial ovarian cancer is the fifth most common malignancy in women and the second leading cause of death due to gynaecological cancer worldwide [1]. The majority of patients are diagnosed at an advanced International Federation of Gynecology and Obstetrics (FIGO) stage due to limitation of screening and the nonspecific nature of symptoms. The 5-year survival rate for women with early pelvic disease is over 70% but less than 30% for those with advanced metastatic disease [2]. Epithelial ovarian carcinomas are histologically categorised into serous (75%), mucinous (10%), endometrioid (10%), clear cell (1%) and undifferentiated (1%) subtypes. Maximal cytoreductive surgery and chemotherapy (carboplatin and paclitaxel) remain the two mainstays of adjuvant therapy, but approximately 70% of patients with advanced disease will relapse despite response to initial treatments [3].

OVARIAN CANCER IMMUNOTHERAPY

Immunotherapy represents an alternative and rational approach for the treatment of cancer, including ovarian cancer. A major function of the immune system is to continually seek out and eliminate cancer cells as they arise in a process referred to as cancer immunosurveillance [4]. Immunosurveillance involves both innate and adaptive immune mechanisms which function complimentarily to promote tumour immunity. Key to the antitumour immune responses is that it can be induced by immunological agents.

Several lines of clinical evidence collectively suggest that the immune system is protective against ovarian cancers and therefore forms the basis of immunotherapy for this disease. This is shown by a number of studies including a representative immunohistochemical analysis (186 advanced-stage ovarian cancers) which showed that 54.8% contained CD3+ T cells and that the presence of intratumoral T cells was associated with a higher 5-year overall survival (OS) rate of patients; 38% for those positive for T cells and 4.5% for those negative for T cells. In addition, patients with tumours containing T cells had a longer progression-free survival (PFS); 22.4 months and 5.8 months respectively [6]. To date, a number of ovarian cancer-associated antigens have been identified, including cancer antigen 125 (CA125) [7], homeobox protein A7 (HOXA7) [8], the cancer/testis antigen NY-ESO-1 [9,10], human epidermal growth factor (HER)-2/neu [11] and recently the P1 antigen [12]. These represent potential targets for therapeutic antibodies in cellular- and/or humoral-mediated antitumour immune responses.

ANTIBODIES AS THERAPEUTIC AGENTS FOR CANCER

Antibodies are glycoproteins composed of two heavy chains and two light chains joined by disulphide bonds, with the antigen-binding site located at the C-terminus and the constant region at the N-terminus. They are excellent anticancer agents by virtue of their high specificity for antigen, stability and easy generation via bioengineering technology. Antibodies can potentially induce tumour cell apoptosis via a number of mechanisms including (1) complement-dependent cytotoxicity (CDC), (2) antibody-dependent cellular cytotoxicity (ADCC), (3) indirect induction of tumour cell death through modulation of antitumour immunity via blockade of immune checkpoint inhibitors and (4) limiting tumour growth by binding to growth receptors, preventing interactions with endogenous ligands and hence inhibiting downstream signalling events.

Here we will introduce recent developments in various antibody-based immunotherapies undergoing clinical trials for ovarian cancer. In addition, we will also shed light on antiglycan antibodies, which are naturally occurring antibodies (NAbs) that recognise exclusively polysaccharide epitopes rather than peptide epitopes localised on proteins and lipid chains.

Catumaxomab

Catumaxomab (Removab) is a monoclonal bispecific antibody approved in 2009 in the European Union for the intraperitoneal treatment of patients with malignant ascites. The antibody has two different antigen-binding sites: one for human epithelial cell adhesion molecule EpCAM (via a heavy and light chain of a rat IgG2b antibody), a type I transmembrane glycoprotein frequently overexpressed in ovarian cancers associated with lower OS [13,14], making EpCAM an attractive target in cancer immunotherapies; and one for human CD3 (via a heavy and light chain of a mouse IgG2a). The rationale of using catumaxomab is to activate and recruit T cells to EpCAM-expressing tumours whilst simultaneously stimulating accessory cells via their Fcγ receptors. The result is tumour cell destruction by ADCC and/or T-cell-mediated cytotoxicity via perforin and granzyme B [15].

Over 90% of ovarian cancer patients have EpCAM overexpressed on tumour cells present in ascites [16]. A phase I/II clinical trial involving 23 ovarian cancer patients with recurrent ascites due to progressive chemoresistant disease showed that treatment with catumaxomab resulted in a highly significant and sustained reduction of ascites including reduced or absent EpCAM-positive tumour cells in the ascites [17]. A phase II/III clinical trial with 258 patients with recurrent chemoresistant adenocarcinoma (ovarian, gastric, breast, pancreas, colon, endometrial) presenting with ascites demonstrated a sevenfold prolongation of the time to the next paracentesis [18]. Catumaxomab, an antibody composed of chains of mouse and rat origin, is expected to induce human anti-mouse antibodies (HAMAs) when administered to patients. Catumaxomab did indeed produce greater clinical benefits in cancer patients who developed HAMAs (median puncture-free survival was 64 versus 30 days for HAMA-positive/-negative ovarian cancer responders) [19]. It is generally well tolerated with most common adverse events being reversible mild-to-moderate nausea and abdominal pain, and therefore it appears to be a promising immunotherapy for ovarian cancer and may be particularly useful for patients presenting with chemotherapy-resistant disease and recurrent ascites.

Abagovomab and oregovomab

Antibodies can function as antigens in the form of 'antiidiotypic antibodies'. Immunisation with a given antigen (x) results in the generation of anti-x antibodies, which can be referred to as Ab1 [20]. Neils Jerne proposed that these antibodies may themselves be immunogenic, and he defined the immunogenic determinants of the antibody as idiotopes. The idiotopes of Ab1 can function as antigen that evoke the generation of antibodies (antiidiotypic). Ab2 are antibodies that result from exposure to Ab1, some of which are antiidiotypic. Since idiotopes are concentrated in the highly variable region of the antigen-binding site, some Ab2 will have idiotopes that effectively mimic the three-dimensional structure of antigen x. Experimental evidence suggests that in some circumstances, exposure to Ab2 may provoke a more effective response than exposure to antigen. These antibodies, in turn, may

Table 4.1 Clinical trials of selected antibody-based immunotherapies for ovarian cancer

Immunotherapies in phase I-III trials (ovarian cancer)

Drug	Proposed mode of action	Antibody	Target antigen	Phase	Indication	No. of patients	Clinical notes	Reference no.
Catumaxomab	Trifunctional bi-specific antibody	Nonhumanised chimeric rat IgG2b/mouse IgG2a	EpCAM	I/II	Recurrent ascites due to progressive chemoresistance	23	Reduced ascites volume and number of EpCAM+ in ascites	17
				II/III	Malignant ascites secondary to epithelial adenocarcinomas	258 (129 ovarian)	Treatment associated with longer median puncture-free survival and median time to next paracentesis	18
Abagovomab	Anti-idiotypic vaccine	Murine IgG1k	CA-125	I	FIGO stages III and IV ovarian cancer	42	Increased number of CA-125-specific CD8+ T cells in some patients	26
				I	FIGO stages I-IV ovarian cancer	36	Increased number of CA-125-specific CD8+ T cells in some patients	62
				Ib/II	Ovarian, tubal and peritoneal cancers	119	68.1% patients developed Ab3 responses, correlating with longer overall survival	25
				III	Ovarian cancer	888	Results pending	27
Oregovomab	Activation of idiotypic network	Murine IgG1	CA-125	II	FIGO stages I-IV ovarian cancer	20	Increased T-cell responses to CA-125 and autologous tumour cells in some patients, correlating with longer survival	30
				II	Recurrent ovarian, tubal and peritoneal adenocarcinoma	13	No overt reduction in tumour burden	32
				Not specified	FIGO stages I-IV ovarian cancer	184	Development of anti-CA-125 antibody (Ab3) responses in some patients	29

Table 4.1 *continued*

Drug	Proposed mode of action	Antibody	Target antigen	Phase	Indication	No. of patients	Clinical notes	Reference no.
				Not specified	FIGO stages I–IV ovarian cancer	75	Development of Ab2 and Ab3 levels in some patients. Evidence that Ab3 mediates antibody-dependent cellular cytotoxicity in some patients.	31
				Not specified	FIGO stages I– to IV ovarian cancer	49	Development of Ab2 and Ab3 levels in some patients, correlating with survival advantage	28
				III	FIGO stages III and IV	375	Oregovomab as a monoimmunotherapy did not improve clinical outcomes	33
Daclizumab	Antiregulatory T cell	Humanised IgG1	CD25	Not specified	Not specified	Not specified	Results pending	35
Ontak	Antiregulatory T cell	N/A (fusion protein of IL-2 and diphtheria toxin)	CD25	I/II	Advanced cancer	4 (2 ovarian)	Treatment associated with reduction in regulatory T cell numbers. Significant drop in CA-125 levels in one patient	37,41
Ipilimumab	Activation of effector T cells	Human IgG1	CTLA-4	I	Pretreated advanced melanoma or ovarian cancer	9 (2 ovarian)	CA-125 level stabilisation (one patient) and reduction (one patient)	43
				I	FIGO stage IV ovarian cancer previously received GVAX	9	Antitumour activity in one patient	44
MDX-1105	Immune checkpoint-inhibitor	IgG4	PD-L1	I	Not specified	207 (17 ovarian)	One partial response, three stable disease	49
CVac	Adoptive transfer of vaccine-primed T cells	Autologous dendritic cell-derived Ab	Mucin1	II	Recurrent advanced ovarian cancer	6	Vaccine-induced restoration of antitumour immunity in two patients	52,53

Adapted from Tse et al (2014) [5]. FIGO, International Federation of Gynecology and Obstetrics.

stimulate the production of Ab3, some of which target the idiotopes of Ab2, and bind to antigen x.

CA125 is a high molecular weight mucin-like glycoprotein overexpressed on the surface of ovarian cancer cells. It is also shed into the bloodstream and is currently the most widely used tumour marker for ovarian cancer. A high level of serum CA125 at ovarian cancer diagnosis frequently indicates widespread peritoneal dissemination, and a continual increase in its value generally indicates disease progression [21,7]. Although CA125 is in clinical use as a tumour marker, its biological function is still poorly understood: some studies suggest that it is involved in cell adhesion, migration, metastasis, invasion and may have immunosuppressive properties [22,23].

Abagovomab (ACA-126) is a murine IgG1k monoclonal antibody (Ab2) with its idiotope imitating CA125 and is currently being investigated as an antiidiotypic vaccine for ovarian cancer. A phase I trial (42 patients with chemotherapy-resistant ovarian cancers; 93% with FIGO stages III-IV; 67% serous histotype) showed that abagovomab induced Ab3 and HAMA responses in all patients, that five of five patients also had detectable CA125-specific interferon gamma (IFN-γ)-producing T cells post vaccination, whereas none were detectable in any subjects prior to treatment, and that abagovomab in 25 patients strongly increased serum levels of IFN-γ, indicative of the induction of Th1 immune responses [24]. A phase Ib/II clinical trial with 119 patients with CA125-positive ovarian, tubal or peritoneal cancers showed that 68.1% of patients who received abagovomab developed Ab3 responses and exhibited significantly longer OS (23.4 vs. 4 months) even when stratified for FIGO stage, type of first-line chemotherapy and the number of previous therapies [25]. The mechanism by which abagovomab exerts its antitumour effect is likely to be ADCC. Such promising data together with the generally well-tolerability of the drug resulted in the initiation of a randomised double-blind placebo-controlled phase III trial involving 888 patients with FIGO stage III/IV ovarian cancer known as the 'Monoclonal antibody Immunotherapy for Malignancies of Ovary by Subcutaneous Abagovomab' (MIMOSA) trial [26]. Whilst abagovomab was shown to be safe and induced measurable immune responses, the study concluded that when the antibody was employed as a maintenance therapy for patients with first remission, it did not prolong relapse-free and OS [27].

Oregovomab (B43.13, OvRex) is a murine monoclonal antibody of IgG1 subclass with high affinity for CA125 (K_D = 1.2 – 10^{10} M^{-1}). It was initially developed as a technetium 99c-labelled antibody for the immunoscintigraphic detection of recurrent ovarian cancer by virtue of its expression of CA125 [28]. However, some patients who received this tumour-imaging agent had an unexpected survival advantage, prompting investigations into the antibody's potential as a therapy for ovarian cancer. Oregovomab evokes anti-CA125 antibody production and elicits tumour-specific T-cell responses rather than directly inhibiting tumour growth or inducing CDC or ADCC by itself.

A trial with 184 patients with ovarian cancer (FIGO stages I-IV) showed that a single treatment of oregovomab caused a rapid reduction in serum levels of CA125 due to the formation of immune complexes, that 26 out of 60 (43%) patients had a greater than threefold increase in anti-CA125 antibody levels, that anti-CA125 antibody responders also had longer survival times compared with nonresponders (22.9 vs. 13.5 months) and that 53% of patients showed an increase in T-cell proliferation in response to CA125, all together suggesting that the generation of humoral and cellular anti-CA125 responses contributes to the clinical benefits of oregovomab treatment [29]. Similarly, a phase II trial with 20 patients with platinum-resistant recurrent ovarian cancer (FIGO stages I-IV) demonstrated an oregovomab-increased T-cell response to CA125 in 39% of patients and to autologous tumour cells in 63%, both associated with longer survival [30]. In another trial with 75 patients with ovarian cancer (FIGO stages I-IV), oregovomab treatment (1-10 infusions) resulted in Ab2 antibody development in 64% and in anti-CA125 antibody development in 24% of the patients [31]. In a retrospective analysis of a previous trial with 44 patients with recurrent ovarian cancer (majority being FIGO stages III-IV), treatment with oregovomab resulted in the development of HAMA in 27 out of 40 patients (67.5%), antiidiotypic antibodies (Ab2) in 76.7% of patients, an increase by more than threefold in the level of anti-CA125 antibodies in 28% of patients and the ability of patients to generate these idiotypic network-related antibodies also correlated with a survival advantage [28]. Unfortunately, such promising clinical benefits of oregovomab were not confirmed in other studies. Although immune responses were observed, no overt tumour burden reduction was observed with oregovomab [32], clinical outcomes were similar to those given placebo [33], and more vigorous immune response were observed with carboplatin-paclitaxel administered in combination with oregovomab than observed with oregovomab in monoimmunotherapy [34].

Daclizumab and Ontak

Daclizumab (Zenapax) is a cell-depleting humanised IgG1 monoclonal antibody specific for CD25 and is currently being evaluated in clinical trials as an immunotherapy for a variety of cancers including ovarian cancer [35]. CD25 is expressed on regulatory T cells and on activated effector T cells. CD25+T cells were reported to be abundant in malignant ascites from previously untreated ovarian cancer patients compared to nonmalignant ascites and were also more abundant in FIGO stages III–IV ovarian cancers than in stages I–II tumours [36]. Moreover, higher tumour infiltration of regulatory T cells correlated with shorter patient survival [37,38], suggesting that regulatory T cells may facilitate ovarian cancer progression. Therefore, strategies which block or transiently deplete these cells may prove useful in treating cancer patients, a concept supported by animal studies whereby systemic removal of CD25+ cells with a cell-depleting monoclonal antibody can elicit potent and durable antitumour responses [39,40]. Whilst awaiting the results from clinical trials of daclizumab in ovarian cancer, data from clinical trials of Ontak, another form of CD25-targeted therapy, are encouraging.

Ontak (denileukin diftitox) is an engineered protein combining IL-2 with diphtheria toxin causing apoptosis of CD25+ cells. It is Food and Drug Administration (FDA) approved for the treatment of cutaneous T-cell leukaemia and currently being investigated as a therapy for other cancer types including metastatic ovarian cancer. In a phase I/II clinical trial with seven patients with advanced adenocarcinomas, including ovarian cancer, Ontak treatment was generally well tolerated, reduced CD3+CD4+CD25+ cells in peripheral blood, increased the number of circulating IFN-γ-producing T cells [36] and significantly reduced blood CA125 level in one patient with FIGO stage IV ovarian cancer associated with the resolution of all lymph node, visceral and bone metastases [41].

Ipilimumab

Ipilimumab (MDX-CTLA-4, Yervoy) is a fully human IgG1 monoclonal antibody. Ipilimumab binds to and blocks the activity of cytotoxic T-lymphocyte-associated antigen 4, CTLA-4, a homologue of CD28 expressed on the surface of T cells upon activation and a key molecule in the downregulation of T-cell activity as a means to limit self-damage. In this sense, CTLA-4 functions as an immune-checkpoint receptor that mediates immune suppression. The use of therapeutic agents to block CTLA-4 function prevents immune inactivation and therefore is a rational approach to evoke effective antitumour immune responses. Ipilimumab was recently approved by the FDA for the treatment of advanced melanoma [42], but a few studies have been conducted in ovarian cancer. One of those, a phase I/II trial with 11 patients with FIGO stage IV ovarian cancers who had previously either received chemotherapy or GVAX [a vaccine product composed of autologous, irradiated tumour cells engineered to secrete the immune stimulatory cytokine, granulocyte macrophage colony-stimulating factor (GM-CSF)] showed that ipilimumab was generally well tolerated with the exception of some grade 3 inflammatory toxicities, and exhibited significant antitumour effects in one ovarian cancer patient who showed a dramatic fall of serum CA125 levels during treatment with a substantial regression of a large hepatic metastasis, mesenteric lymph nodes and an omental cake, resulting in pain and ascites reduction. Four other patients had stabilisation of disease as assessed by blood CA125 levels and imaging [43,44].

CURRENT STATE OF IMMUNOTHERAPY IN OVARIAN CANCER

It is still unclear whether immunotherapy, both vaccine- and antibody-based, has the potential to be incorporated into treatment regimens against ovarian cancer. For the former, a study with 12 patients with relapsed epithelial ovarian cancer has recently been performed to increase the NY-ESO-1 vaccine efficacy [45]. This phase I dose-escalation trial of decitabine (a DNA methyltransferase inhibitor), as an addition to NY-ESO-1 vaccine and doxorubicin liposome (doxorubicin) chemotherapy, showed increased NY-ESO-1 serum antibodies and T-cell responses in the majority of patients (disease stabilisation or partial clinical response in 6 out of 10 evaluable patients), warranting further evaluation of similar combinatorial chemoimmunotherapy regimens in epithelial ovarian cancer. For the latter, an increasing number of antibody-based immunotherapeutics have reached the clinical trial stage over the past decade. Whilst catumaxomab, abagovomab and oregovomab have already reached phase III, many other new antibody-based treatments have just entered phase I and II clinical trials. Catumaxomab particularly shows promise and was recently approved by the European Community for the treatment of malignant ascites. Results from larger trials of this antibody are greatly anticipated. Abagovomab and oregovomab, both of which appeared promising based on early clinical trials, have been largely disappointing in recent phase III trials with no overt antitumour efficacy reported. In recent years, immune-checkpoint inhibitors such as ipilimumab, MDX-1105 and MDX-1106, have emerged as candidates for cancer immunotherapy but only a few small clinical trials for ovarian cancer have been conducted so far.

MDX-1105 and MDX-1106, contrary to ipilimumab, target the PD-1/PD-L1 axis. In contrast to CTLA-4, the main function of which is to regulate the activation of naive T cells, PD-1 (programmed cell death 1) predominantly restrains the activity of effector T cells within peripheral tissues (e.g. sites of chronic inflammation, infection or cancer) to limit autoimmunity [46]. Interaction of PD-1 with its ligand, PD-1 ligand 1 (PD-L1), inhibits T-cell proliferation, survival and effector functions, induces apoptosis of antigen-specific T cells, promotes the conversion of CD4+ T cells to regulatory T cells and induces tumour resistance to cytotoxic T-cell killing [47]. Therefore, blockade of the PD-1/PD-L1 axis could potentially enhance the strength of antitumour immunity, with the goal to produce durable clinical responses. In ovarian cancer, PD-L1 expression has been shown to be an independent factor for poor prognosis [48]. The results indicate that the PD-1/PD-L1 axis is involved in immune evasion in ovarian cancer, and that blockade of this immune checkpoint pathway may unleash the potential of antitumour immunity to mediate tumour regression.

MDX-1105 (BMS-936559) is a fully human IgG4 monoclonal antibody with high affinity for PD-L1. It inhibits the binding of PD-L1 to PD-1, and is a noncell-depleting antibody. A phase I clinical trial with 207 patients with a variety of cancer types reported encouraging results [49]. In the ovarian cancer arm, 1 of 17 patients (6%) had a partial response (defined as at least a 30% decrease in the sum of the largest diameter of target lesions) and 3 (18%) had stable disease lasting over 24 weeks.

MDX-1106 (BMS-936558) is also a fully human IgG4-blocking monoclonal antibody that is directed against PD-1. To date, there have been two phase I clinical trials which investigated the safety and antitumour activity of this antibody, although neither recruited ovarian cancer patients [50,51]. However, results from other cancer types are showing promise and inclusion of ovarian cancer patients in future trials is warranted.

A promising advance can be highlighted by a recent report of George Coukos and coworkers [52]. They demonstrated that an autologous dendritic cell-derived antibody directed against mucin1 (CVac), a glycoprotein highly overexpressed in ovarian cancer, triggered an antitumour response in ovarian cancer patients who were unresponsive to existing treatments. This two-step personalised immunotherapy treatment showed a vaccine-induced restoration of antitumour immunity in these patients with an improved median PFS at the time of the second remission. A respective phase II clinical trial (CAN-003) has just been completed and was presented at the American Society of Clinical Oncology-Meeting in 2014 [53]. This study was the first immunotherapy trial showing a positive survival result for ovarian cancer patients by extending their PFS from the treatment with CVac. Mucin1 is an ideal target for immunotherapy as it is a glycoprotein which is overexpressed in many adenocarcinomas including ovarian cancers (83%). Patients receiving CVac showed no benefit in PFS at the time of their first relapse ($P = 0.69$). However, an improved PFS was seen at the time of their second relapse with a median PFS without immunotherapy of 4.9 months compared to over 12.9 months with immunotherapy (endpoint not yet reached); $P = 0.04$; hazard ratio 0.329. These results suggest that survival effects from immunotherapy may take longer than previously estimated and caution has to be taken to downplay overoptimistic interpretation of early trial results.

CRITICAL CONSIDERATIONS OF IMMUNOTHERAPY AND LESSONS LEARNT

For the field of immunotherapy research to move forward, it is important to consider the limiting factors of clinical trials in order to improve the design of future studies.

One limitation common to almost all cancer clinical trials is that the patients already have advanced disease. This is a major issue especially for immunotherapy because the ability to initiate an immune response, or its magnitude, is limited by the extent of disease burden, the suppressive effect of the tumour microenvironment and the multiple layers of immunological tolerance mechanisms (e.g. regulatory T cells) which keep the immune response in check. As a consequence, immune-based therapies are more likely to be effective in patients with low volume disease such as earlier stage cancers or immediately after cytoreductive treatment with minimal residual disease.

A consideration not to be overlooked is whether immunotherapies are offered as monotherapy or as an adjunct therapy. Realistically, if immunotherapy is to be applied to ovarian cancer treatment regimens in the short-to-medium term, it would be as an adjunct therapy rather than as a frontline monotherapy. Future clinical trials should investigate the synergistic potential of immune-modulating agents with established chemotherapies. Indeed, oregovomab was recently investigated as a combination therapy with standard carboplatin–paclitaxel in a phase II clinical trial, and stronger immune responses were measured than those reported in a previous monoimmunotherapy protocol [34]. Chemoimmunotherapy is appealing not only because chemotherapies directly induce apoptosis of tumour cells and result in the release of antigen to drive immune responses, but they often also disrupt essential immune regulatory mechanisms that limit the development of immunity, an increasingly appreciated attribute [54]. An ideal combination of chemoimmunotherapy would be one where both agents have minimal overlapping toxicities, work via independent mechanisms but have additive or synergistic antitumour effects. A successful example of this approach is the combination of fludarabine, cyclophosphamide and rituximab for chronic lymphocytic leukaemia. The addition of rituximab to the chemotherapies increased the rate of complete remission and OS [55]. However, it is critical to optimise the dosage, sequence and timing of administering each drug as all these parameters could impact on the outcome.

Another point to consider in the design of future clinical trials is to acknowledge that ovarian cancer is a heterogeneous disease with four major histological subtypes, each of which has distinct genetic profiles which may affect the ability and/or magnitude of immune responses evoked by an immunotherapy. The heterogeneity of ovarian cancer can be further highlighted by differences in the antiglycan antibody profiles in serum and ascites of patients with various histotypes (discussed in more detail below). Therefore, it may be necessary to conduct clinical trials on more homogenous populations; e.g. serous cancer patients only, to have greater power to detect potential clinical efficacy. Pooling patients into a single cohort may reduce the sensitivity to detect clinical benefits to certain histotypes. The importance of stratifying treatment based on histotype is supported by recent evidence of contrasting clinical outcomes in mucinous and serous ovarian cancers when treated with platinum-based chemotherapy [56]; these two histotypes may be distinct entities, and investigations are underway to determine how each could be managed best.

Naturally occurring antiglycan antibodies: new players in ovarian cancer diagnosis and therapy?

NAbs are immunoglobulins predominantly of IgM class which are secreted by B1 B cells in the absence of external antigen stimulation. They play an important role in protection against infectious material, removal of cellular waste and in limiting chronic inflammation [57]. NAbs bind to oligosaccharides with low affinity and are oligoreactive. There is emerging evidence that these antibodies play an important role in cancer immunosurveillance. It was shown that tumour-specific NAbs exist in both healthy individuals and cancer patients, and can recognise and eliminate intact tumour cells via CDC [58].

Recently, our group reported an intriguing relationship between ovarian cancer, carbohydrate antigens and antiglycan antibodies. Using a printed glycan array, we demonstrated that ovarian cancer patients had significantly different levels of antibodies to a variety of glycans including several established tumour-associated carbohydrate antigens as compared to healthy women [59–61]. This was recently confirmed by our in-house developed suspension glycan array. In addition, it demonstrated that the ability of antiglycan antibodies to discriminate between the two groups was due to IgM rather than IgG in most cases and was also patient cohort independent [12]. The glycan with the most significant discriminatory ability was P1, a member of the P blood group antigens. P1 is covalently attached to ceramide to form a glycosphingolipid; glycosphingolipids are essential constituents of mammalian cell membranes. We recently reported that P1 is expressed on the surface of ovarian cancer cell lines as well as ovarian cancer tissue, and that it is functionally related to cell migration [12]. As such, P1 is a potential biomarker for ovarian cancer, and may be a rational target for immunotherapies.

An important lesson learnt in recent years is not to become overly excited with novel drugs that show particular promise in phase I and/or II clinical trials because quite often they fail to meet the high expectations in phase III studies. Although these results seem disappointing, it is important for research into immunotherapy for ovarian cancer, in combination with chemotherapy, to continue because there are glimpses of efficacy in some patients from initial studies. We need to think critically about the reasons for this, and design future clinical trials accordingly.

CONCLUSION

A wide range of immune-modulating approaches are currently being evaluated for the treatment of ovarian cancer. As the results of clinical trials of the discussed antibody-based immunotherapies are inconsistent, it is still too early to conclude if these drugs will be incorporated into treatment regimens against ovarian cancer. Furthermore, their true potential may lie within being strategically employed in chemoimmunotherapy regimens.

Key points for clinical practice

- Various forms of immunotherapy continue to be evaluated in clinical trials for ovarian cancer, especially within the context of advanced disease and/or relapse.
- It is currently too early to tell whether or not immunotherapy will be utilised in future treatment regimens for ovarian cancer, but research in this field is active.
- The optimal timing and scheduling of immunotherapy together with conventional therapies need to be established in future clinical trials.
- It is important to acknowledge that ovarian cancer is a heterogeneous disease, and therefore the different histotypes may require different treatment modalities. Antiglycan antibodies are NAbs and might be a new class of antibodies which could be used for immunotherapy.

REFERENCES

1. Jemal A, Bray F, Center MM, et al. Global cancer statistics. CA Cancer J Clin 2011; 61:69–90.
2. Siegel R, Naishadham D, Jemal A. Cancer statistics, 2012. CA Cancer J Clin 2012; 62:10–29.
3. Ushijima K. Treatment for recurrent ovarian cancer-at first relapse. J Oncol 2010; 2010:497429.
4. Smyth MJ, Dunn GP, Schreiber RD. Cancer immunosurveillance and immunoediting: the roles of immunity in suppressing tumor development and shaping tumor immunogenicity. Adv Immunol 2006; 90:1–50.
5. Tse BW, Collins A, Oehler MK, et al. Antibody-based immunotherapy for ovarian cancer: where are we at? Ann Oncol 2014; 25:322–331.
6. Zhang L, Conejo-Garcia JR, Katsaros D, et al. Intratumoral T cells, recurrence, and survival in epithelial ovarian cancer. N Engl J Med 2003; 348:203–213.
7. Bast RC, Jr. CA 125 and the detection of recurrent ovarian cancer: a reasonably accurate biomarker for a difficult disease. Cancer 2010; 116:2850–2853.
8. Naora H, Montz FJ, Chai CY, et al. Aberrant expression of homeobox gene HOXA7 is associated with mullerian-like differentiation of epithelial ovarian tumors and the generation of a specific autologous antibody response. Proc Natl Acad Sci U S A 2001; 98:15209–15214.
9. Odunsi K, Jungbluth AA, Stockert E, et al. NY-ESO-1 and LAGE-1 cancer-testis antigens are potential targets for immunotherapy in epithelial ovarian cancer. Cancer Res 2003; 63:6076–6083.
10. Odunsi K, Matsuzaki J, Karbach J, et al. Efficacy of vaccination with recombinant vaccinia and fowlpox vectors expressing NY-ESO-1 antigen in ovarian cancer and melanoma patients. Proc Natl Acad Sci U S A 2012; 109:5797–5802.
11. Camilleri-Broet S, Hardy-Bessard AC, Le Tourneau A, et al. HER-2 overexpression is an independent marker of poor prognosis of advanced primary ovarian carcinoma: a multicenter study of the GINECO group. Ann Oncol 2004; 15:104–112.
12. Jacob F, Anugraham M, Pochechueva T, et al. The glycosphingolipid P1 is an ovarian cancer-associated carbohydrate antigen involved in migration. Br J Cancer 2014; 111:1634–1645.
13. Spizzo G, Went P, Dirnhofer S, et al. Overexpression of epithelial cell adhesion molecule (Ep-CAM) is an independent prognostic marker for reduced survival of patients with epithelial ovarian cancer. Gynecol Oncol 2006; 103:483–488.
14. Heinzelmann-Schwarz VA, Gardiner-Garden M, Henshall SM, et al. Overexpression of the cell adhesion molecules DDR1, Claudin 3, and Ep-CAM in metaplastic ovarian epithelium and ovarian cancer. Clin Cancer Res 2004; 10:4427–4436.
15. Seimetz D, Lindhofer H, Bokemeyer C. Development and approval of the trifunctional antibody catumaxomab (anti-EpCAM x anti-CD3) as a targeted cancer immunotherapy. Cancer Treat Rev 2010; 36:458–467.
16. Diaz-Arias AA, Loy TS, Bickel JT, et al. Utility of BER-EP4 in the diagnosis of adenocarcinoma in effusions: an immunocytochemical study of 232 cases. Diagn Cytopathol 1993; 9:516–521.
17. Burges A, Wimberger P, Kumper C, et al. Effective relief of malignant ascites in patients with advanced ovarian cancer by a trifunctional anti-EpCAM x anti-CD3 antibody: a phase I/II study. Clin Cancer Res 2007; 13:3899–3905.
18. Heiss MM, Murawa P, Koralewski P, et al. The trifunctional antibody catumaxomab for the treatment of malignant ascites due to epithelial cancer: results of a prospective randomized phase II/III trial. Int J Cancer 2010; 127:2209–2221.
19. Ott MG, Marme F, Moldenhauer G, et al. Humoral response to catumaxomab correlates with clinical outcome: results of the pivotal phase II/III study in patients with malignant ascites. Int J Cancer 2012; 130:2195–2203.
20. Jerne NK. Clonal selection in a lymphocyte network. Soc Gen Physiol Ser 1974; 29:39–48.
21. Rustin GJ, Marples M, Nelstrop AE, et al. Use of CA-125 to define progression of ovarian cancer in patients with persistently elevated levels. J Clin Oncol 2001; 19:4054–4057.
22. Gubbels JA, Belisle J, Onda M, et al. Mesothelin-MUC16 binding is a high affinity, N-glycan dependent interaction that facilitates peritoneal metastasis of ovarian tumors. Mol Cancer 2006; 5:50.
23. Patankar MS, Jing Y, Morrison JC, et al. Potent suppression of natural killer cell response mediated by the ovarian tumor marker CA125. Gynecol Oncol 2005; 99:704–713.
24. Sabbatini P, Dupont J, Aghajanian C, et al. Phase I study of abagovomab in patients with epithelial ovarian, fallopian tube, or primary peritoneal cancer. Clin Cancer Res 2006; 12:5503–5510.

25. Reinartz S, Kohler S, Schlebusch H, et al. Vaccination of patients with advanced ovarian carcinoma with the anti-idiotype ACA125: immunological response and survival (phase Ib/II). Clin Cancer Res 2004; 10:1580–1587.

26. Sabbatini P, Berek JS, Casada A, et al. Abagovomab maintenance therapy in patients with epithelial ovarian cancer after complete response (CR) post-first-line chemotherapy (FLCT): preliminary results of the randomized, double-blind, placebo-controlled, multicenter MIMOSA trial. J Clin Oncol 2010; 28;15 Suppl:5036.

27. Sabbatini P, Harter P, Scambia G, et al. Abagovomab as maintenance therapy in patients with epithelial ovarian cancer: a phase III trial of the AGO OVAR, COGI, GINECO, and GEICO––the MIMOSA study. J Clin Oncol 2013; 31:1554–1561.

28. Mobus VJ, Baum RP, Bolle M, et al. Immune responses to murine monoclonal antibody-B43.13 correlate with prolonged survival of women with recurrent ovarian cancer. Am J Obstet Gynecol 2003; 189:28–36.

29. Noujaim AA, Schultes BC, Baum RP, et al. Induction of CA125-specific B and T cell responses in patients injected with MAb-B43.13––evidence for antibody-mediated antigen-processing and presentation of CA125 in vivo. Cancer Biother Radiopharm 2001; 16:187–203.

30. Gordon AN, Schultes BC, Gallion H, et al. CA125- and tumor-specific T-cell responses correlate with prolonged survival in oregovomab-treated recurrent ovarian cancer patients. Gynecol Oncol 2004; 94:340–351.

31. Schultes BC, Baum RP, Niesen A, et al. Anti-idiotype induction therapy: anti-CA125 antibodies (Ab3) mediated tumor killing in patients treated with Ovarex mAb B43.13 (Ab1). Cancer Immunol Immunother 1998; 46:201–212.

32. Ehlen TG, Hoskins PJ, Miller D, et al. A pilot phase 2 study of oregovomab murine monoclonal antibody to CA125 as an immunotherapeutic agent for recurrent ovarian cancer. Int J Gynecol Cancer 2005; 15:1023–1034.

33. Berek J, Taylor P, McGuire W, et al. Oregovomab maintenance monoimmunotherapy does not improve outcomes in advanced ovarian cancer. J Clin Oncol 2009; 27:418–425.

34. Braly P, Nicodemus CF, Chu C, et al. The immune adjuvant properties of front-line carboplatin-paclitaxel: a randomized phase 2 study of alternative schedules of intravenous oregovomab chemoimmunotherapy in advanced ovarian cancer. J Immunother 2009; 32:54–65.

35. Vasievich EA, Huang L. The suppressive tumor microenvironment: a challenge in cancer immunotherapy. Mol Pharm 2011; 8:635-641.

36. Barnett B, Kryczek I, Cheng P, et al. Regulatory T cells in ovarian cancer: biology and therapeutic potential. Am J Reprod Immunol 2005; 54:369–377.

37. Barnett JC, Bean SM, Whitaker RS, et al. Ovarian cancer tumor infiltrating T-regulatory (T(reg)) cells are associated with a metastatic phenotype. Gynecol Oncol 2010; 116:556–562.

38. Sato E, Olson SH, Ahn J, et al. Intraepithelial CD8+ tumor-infiltrating lymphocytes and a high CD8+/regulatory T cell ratio are associated with favorable prognosis in ovarian cancer. Proc Natl Acad Sci U S A 2005; 102:18538–18543.

39. Shimizu J, Yamazaki S, Sakaguchi S. Induction of tumor immunity by removing CD25+CD4+ T cells: a common basis between tumor immunity and autoimmunity. J Immunol 1999; 163:5211–5218.

40. Tien AH, Xu L, Helgason CD. Altered immunity accompanies disease progression in a mouse model of prostate dysplasia. Cancer Res 2005; 65:2947–2955.

41. Barnett B, Kryczek I, Cheng P, et al. Regulatory T cells in ovarian cancer: biology and therapeutic potential. Am J Reprod Immunol 2005;54:369-377.

42. Sondak VK, Smalley KS, Kudchadkar R, et al. Ipilimumab. Nat Rev Drug Discov 2011; 10:411–412.

43. Hodi FS, Mihm MC, Soiffer RJ, et al. Biologic activity of cytotoxic T lymphocyte-associated antigen 4 antibody blockade in previously vaccinated metastatic melanoma and ovarian carcinoma patients. Proc Natl Acad Sci U S A 2003; 100:4712–4717.

44. Hodi FS, Butler M, Oble DA, et al. Immunologic and clinical effects of antibody blockade of cytotoxic T lymphocyte-associated antigen 4 in previously vaccinated cancer patients. Proc Natl Acad Sci U S A 2008; 105:3005–3010.

45. Odunsi K, Matsuzaki J, James SR, et al. Epigenetic potentiation of NY-ESO-1 vaccine therapy in human ovarian cancer. Cancer Immunol Res 2014; 2:37–49.

46. Pardoll DM. The blockade of immune checkpoints in cancer immunotherapy. Nat Rev Cancer 2012; 12:252–264.

47. Zitvogel L, Kroemer G. Targeting PD-1/PD-L1 interactions for cancer immunotherapy. Oncoimmunology 2012; 1:1-3.
48. Hamanishi J, Mandai M, Iwasaki M, et al. Programmed cell death 1 ligand 1 and tumor-infiltrating CD8+ T lymphocytes are prognostic factors of human ovarian cancer. Proc Natl Acad Sci U S A 2007; 104:3360–3365.
49. Brahmer JR, Tykodi SS, Chow LQ, et al. Safety and activity of anti-PD-L1 antibody in patients with advanced cancer. N Engl J Med 2012; 366:2455–2465.
50. Brahmer JR, Drake CG, Wollner I, et al. Phase I study of single-agent anti-programmed death-1 (MDX-1106) in refractory solid tumors: safety, clinical activity, pharmacodynamics, and immunologic correlates. J Clin Oncol 2010; 28:3167–3175.
51. Topalian SL, Hodi FS, Brahmer JR, et al. Safety, activity, and immune correlates of anti-PD-1 antibody in cancer. N Engl J Med 2012; 366:2443–2454.
52. Kandalaft LE, Powell DJ, Jr., Chiang CL, et al. Autologous lysate-pulsed dendritic cell vaccination followed by adoptive transfer of vaccine-primed ex vivo co-stimulated T cells in recurrent ovarian cancer. Oncoimmunology. 2013; 2:e22664.
53. Gray HJ, Gargosky SE, CAN-003 Study Team. Progression-free survival in ovarian cancer patients in second remission with mucin-1 autologous dendritic cell therapy. J Clin Oncol 2014; 32;15 Suppl:5504.
54. Emens LA. Chemotherapy and tumor immunity: an unexpected collaboration. Front Biosci 2008; 13:249–257.
55. Tam CS, Keating MJ. Chemoimmunotherapy of chronic lymphocytic leukemia. Nat Rev Clin Oncol 2010; 7:521–532.
56. Naik JD, Seligmann J, Perren TJ. Mucinous tumours of the ovary. J Clin Pathol 2012; 65:580–584.
57. Schwartz-Albiez R, Monteiro RC, Rodriguez M, et al. Natural antibodies, intravenous immunoglobulin and their role in autoimmunity, cancer and inflammation. Clin Exp Immunol 2009; 158 Suppl 1:43–50.
58. Brandlein S, Pohle T, Ruoff N, et al. Natural IgM antibodies and immunosurveillance mechanisms against epithelial cancer cells in humans. Cancer Res 2003; 63:7995–8005.
59. Jacob F, Goldstein DR, Bovin NV, et al. Serum antiglycan antibody detection of nonmucinous ovarian cancers by using a printed glycan array. Int J Cancer 2012; 130:138–146.
60. Pochechueva T, Jacob F, Fedier A, et al. Tumor-associated glycans and their role in gynecological cancers: accelerating translational research by novel high-throughput approaches. Metabolites 2012; 2:913–939.
61. Pochechueva T, Jacob F, Goldstein DR, et al. Comparison of printed glycan array, suspension array and ELISA in the detection of human anti-glycan antibodies. Glycoconj J 2011; 28:507–517.
62. Pfisterer J, du Bois A, Sehouli J, et al. The anti-idiotypic antibody abagovomab in patients with recurrent ovarian cancer. A phase I trial of the AGO-OVAR. Ann Oncol 2006; 17:1568–1577.

Chapter 5

The obese woman in late pregnancy and labour

Amy O'Higgins, Michael J Turner

INTRODUCTION

Adults are classified as obese based on the World Health Organization (WHO) categorisation of a body mass index (BMI) >29.9 kg/m² (**Table 5.1**). Maternal obesity has emerged as one of the major challenges in obstetrics worldwide because it is common, it is associated with an increase in pregnancy complications and interventions, it presents

Classification	BMI (kg/m²)	
	Cut-off points	**Additional cut-off points**
Underweight	<18.50	<18.50
Severe thinness	<16.00	<16.00
Moderate thinness	16.00–16.99	16.00–16.99
Mild thinness	17.00–18.49	17.00–18.49
Normal range	18.50–24.99	18.50–22.99
		23.00–24.99
Overweight	≥25.00	≥25.00
Pre-obese	25.00–29.99	25.00–27.49
		27.50–29.99
Obese	≥30.00	≥30.00
Obese class I	30.00–34.99	30.00–32.49
		32.50–34.99
Obese class II	35.00–39.99	35.00–37.49
		37.50–39.99
Obese class III	≥40.00	≥40.00

Table 5.1 World Health Organization body mass index categorisation

BMI, body mass index.

Amy O'Higgins MRCPI, UCD Centre for Human Reproduction, Coombe Women and Infants University Hospital, Dublin, Ireland

Michael J Turner MAO FRCPI FRCOG, UCD Centre for Human Reproduction, Coombe Women and Infants University Hospital, Dublin, Ireland. Email: michael.turner@ucd.ie (for correspondence)

Table 5.2 Clinical outcomes associated with maternal obesity in a large meta-analysis	
Maternal	Emergency caesarean section (CS) rate
	Total CS rate
	Average length of hospital stay
	Haemorrhage
	Infection
	Induction of labour
	Oxytocin usage
	Epidural analgesia
	Instrumental vaginal delivery
Fetal	Delivery <37 weeks' gestation
	Delivery <32 weeks' gestation
	Neonatal intensive care admissions
	Low Apgar score at 5 minutes
	High birth weight

clinical technical challenges, it is associated with increased healthcare costs and potentially it carries lifelong consequences for the woman and her offspring (**Table 5.2**) [1–4].

Although BMI is only a surrogate marker of adiposity and has its limitations, it is practical and inexpensive to calculate the BMI based on the measurement of a woman's weight and height in early pregnancy [5]. Despite the clinical importance of calculating BMI accurately, it is a concern that many maternity services do not measure and record weight and height at the first antenatal visit, or continue to calculate BMI based on a woman's self-reported weight and height [5,6]. Classification based on self-reporting leads to BMI miscategorisation in 22% of cases and to the diagnosis of obesity being missed in 5% [5–6]. Contrary to earlier beliefs, maternal weight does not usually increase in the first trimester and the baseline BMI during pregnancy can be calculated accurately up to 18–20 weeks' gestation [6]. Whilst there is epidemiological evidence that obesity rates in women of child-bearing age have increased in wealthy countries, there is a paucity of data on obesity trends in pregnant women. In Dublin, about one in six women booking for antenatal care is obese and nearly one in 50 is morbidly obese [2].

MATERNAL OBESITY AND MATERNAL COMPLICATIONS

Gestational diabetes mellitus

Maternal obesity has been associated with an increase in antenatal complications, with the strongest evidence supporting an association with gestational diabetes mellitus (GDM). Indeed, obesity is one of the indications for selective screening at 24–28 weeks' gestation with an oral glucose tolerance test [2]. In one study, GDM was diagnosed in 5.5% of women with mild obesity and 11.5% of women with moderate-to-severe obesity compared with 2.3% in women with a normal BMI [7]. It has also been recommended that women who are more obese should be screened early in pregnancy for GDM because they may have undiagnosed type 2 diabetes mellitus (T2DM) prepregnancy.

Furthermore, the development and implementation of clinical guidelines and a lowering of the diagnostic criteria have led to an increase in the number of obese women diagnosed with GDM. Failure to screen an obese woman for GDM may increase the risk of the delivery being complicated by fetal macrosomia, shoulder dystocia and a brachial plexus injury. The diagnosis of GDM in the obese woman is also an opportunity for the obstetrician to put in place lifestyle interventions that may improve maternal glycaemic control which, if sustained, may prevent or defer the development of T2DM later in a woman's life.

Hyptertensive disorders

Maternal obesity is associated with an increase in hypertensive disorders during pregnancy [8]. If obesity is associated with pre-eclampsia, this, in turn, may require obstetric intervention to deliver the woman early. A practical consideration is that obese women usually need a large cuff for the measurement of their blood pressure (BP) using a manual aneroid sphygmomanometer if their mid-arm circumference is >33 cm [8]. The use of an inappropriately sized cuff may lead to overdiagnosis of hypertension in obese women and thus, an unnecessary increase in investigations, hospital admissions and obstetric interventions. Inaccurate measurement of BP may also have led to the risk of hypertensive disorders being overestimated in large retrospective epidemiological studies on the risks of maternal obesity.

Venous thromboembolism

The incidence of venous thromboembolism (VTE) during pregnancy is estimated at 5–12 per 10,000 pregnancies and is distributed equally in each trimester [9]. VTE is important because pulmonary embolism is a leading cause of maternal mortality in the developed world and is potentially preventable [10]. A recent seminar reported that a maternal BMI >29.9 kg/m^2 was associated with an increased risk [odds ratio (OR) 1.8 95% confidence interval (CI) 1.3–2.4] of antepartum and postpartum VTE [9].

In an American inpatient sample, maternal obesity carried an increased risk (OR 4.5) of VTE [10]. The risk factor with the highest OR (51.8) for VTE was thrombophilia. The association between maternal obesity alone and VTE is weak. If there is an increased risk, we do not know at what level or category of BMI the increase occurs, nor do we know whether any association is due to obesity alone, or whether it is due to comorbidities or confounding variables, such as caesarean section (CS). Any effect of obesity on VTE risk is strongly influenced by immobilisation in hospital [11].

It is standard practice in developed countries to use thromboprophylaxis for all women delivered by CS. However, the dose of thromboprophylaxis using preloaded syringes of low molecular weight heparin (LMWH) should be weight based. In 1995, the Royal College of Obstetricians and Gynaecologists (RCOG) recommended selective thromboprophylaxis post-CS, but the recommendations were implemented in only one fifth of the cases [12]. It now recommends that all women undergoing emergency CS and all obese women undergoing emergency or elective CS should receive heparin prophylaxis for at least 7 days postnatal. The use of thromboprophylaxis for CS is widespread in Europe [12]. In contrast, routine thromboprophylaxis after CS is not recommended in the United States. A systematic review of 64 studies reported a 2% frequency of significant bleeding with LMWH, including wound haematoma [12]. There is a consensus, however, that obese women undergoing CS should receive thromboprophylaxis.

The RCOG recommends that women who are morbidly obese (BMI >39.9 kg/m^2) should receive thromboprophylaxis irrespective of the mode of delivery. A VTE risk assessment should be undertaken in morbidly obese women at their first antenatal visit. It should be repeated if there are pregnancy complications, especially those resulting in immobilisation, and again repeated before the woman is discharged postpartum. The majority of VTEs occur after a vaginal delivery; therefore, it is important that any risk assessment is not confined to women post-CS. The pharmacokinetics of LMWH change during pregnancy and dosage should be based on weight at the first visit, not BMI. The doses should be increased for all women with a booking weight >90 kg, but some units prefer to give half the recommended daily dose twice daily for women >90 kg to reduce complications. The recommended doses for women who are obese are not, however, evidence based. For tinzaparin, the dose may need to be reduced if the creatinine clearance is <20 mL/min.

Urinary incontinence

Obese women are at increased risk of both anal and urinary incontinence which has been attributed to pelvic floor trauma at childbirth [13]. However, in a large (n = 210,678) national study of primiparous women who delivered vaginally in Sweden, obesity was associated with a decreased risk of third/fourth perineal tears [13]. Obesity was also associated with an increased risk of first- and second-degree perineal tears. The main risk factor associated with a third/fourth-degree tear was an instrumental delivery. The authors speculated as to why obese women were, contrary to expectations, less likely to have a third/fourth-degree tear. However, visualisation and examination of the perineum in the obese woman may be restricted and one possibility, not considered, was that the extent of the tear may have been underestimated in obese women. This would explain the increase in the first/second-degree tears in obese women and highlights the need to undertake a thorough pelvic examination in the obese woman particularly after an instrumental vaginal delivery.

Caesarean section

A number of reviews have shown that obese women are nearly twice as likely to be delivered by CS and that variations in obesity rates may explain, in part, variations in CS rates nationally and internationally [14]. In a prospective observational study, obese primigravidas were more likely to have an emergency CS and obese multigravidas were more likely to have an elective CS compared with nonobese women [14]. The obese multigravidas who had an elective CS often had an emergency CS in a previous pregnancy.

In a study of 8580 secundipara at term after a previous CS, 78.5% (n = 6718) underwent a trial of labour [15]. After adjustment for confounding factors, maternal BMI correlated negatively with the rate of successful vaginal birth after caesarean (VBAC), but not with the rate of uterine scar separation. In a study of 510 women attempting a trial of labour, increasing prepregnancy BMI and weight gain between a first and second pregnancy reduced the VBAC rate after a single low transverse CS [16]. Thus, after a primary CS, women should optimise their weight and BMI if they want to improve their chances of a successful VBAC in subsequent pregnancies.

The risk of CS in obese women will be influenced by the overall CS rate in any hospital, but up to half of women who are morbidly obese may end up being delivered by CS, although the fetal benefits remain uncertain. Given the surgical and anaesthetic challenges of a CS in the morbidly obese women, this raises a clinical dilemma in individual cases as to whether an elective CS supervised by senior staff is a safer option for the woman rather than an emergency CS which may occur out-of-hours when staff resources are reduced.

Maternal obesity has been associated with an increased risk of both infection and haemorrhage. However, these associations may be a reflection of the increase in interventions, particularly CS in labour. In view of the association with postpartum haemorrhage, it is important to establish good intravenous access early in labour, which may also be advantageous in the obese women who require regional anaesthesia for labour or delivery.

Induction of labour

Obese women are more likely to have labour induced than nonobese, in part, because they are more likely to require elective delivery for medical complications such as GDM or hypertension [17]. They are also more likely to have labour induced postdates which may be explained by the association of female obesity with polycystic ovarian syndrome and an irregular menstrual cycle. Obese women should be offered sonographic dating of their pregnancy at the first prenatal visit so that spurious postdate inductions are avoided.

In a study of 2000 women, induction of labour in obese primigravidas was associated with an increase in interventions such as epidural analgesia, fetal blood sampling and emergency CS [17]. In contrast, induction of labour in obese multigravidas was not only less common, but also was not associated with an increase in other interventions compared with nonobese multigravidas. Thus, the decision to induce labour in an obese primigravida should only be made for strict obstetric indications and should not be based solely on the ultrasound prediction of a large baby.

There is also evidence that maternal obesity is associated with an increase in both dystocia and fetal distress in the first stage of labour, particularly in primigravidas, which leads to the reported increase in emergency CSs [14,18]. In a study of 4341 women in spontaneous labour, 25.5% were obese. Oxytocin augmentation was used for 60.4% of deliveries [18]. Compared with normal women, women with mild obesity were 2.2 times more likely to require a CS for fetal distress and 1.6 times more likely to require a CS for dystocia. Women with moderate/severe obesity were 4.4 times more likely to require a CS for fetal distress and 3.3 times more likely to require a CS for dystocia. The increase in dystocia in obese women is associated with an increased usage of oxytocin augmentation. This may be due to differences in the pharmacokinetics of oxytocin in obese women [19].

In obese women, it is often technically easier to monitor the electronic fetal heart rate using a scalp electrode rather than an abdominal transducer. If the heart trace shows suspected fetal distress, many maternity units use fetal blood sampling to avoid a CS for a false positive diagnosis [18]. In the obese woman, this too is more challenging and may require a longer than usual amnioscope.

Bariatric surgery

The number of morbidly obese women presenting for antenatal care who have had bariatric surgery to lose weight is increasing [20]. The literature is limited but suggests that women who had the surgery are less likely to develop hypertension, GDM and macrosomia than similar women who have not had surgery. The decrease in GDM and macrosomia has been attributed to malabsorption and it is advisable that this group of high-risk women is also monitored closely for nutritional deficiencies [20]. Previous bariatric surgery has been associated with an increased risk of premature rupture of the membranes but not preterm delivery [20]. Following bariatric surgery, guidelines recommend that a woman waits 12–24 months before conceiving in order to avoid fetal complications due to rapid maternal weight loss and to allow the woman to achieve her weight loss goals. Women who have had bariatric surgery using a band should be reviewed by their surgeon antenatally because adjustment may be necessary [3]. Whilst many of these women may have previously been delivered by CS, a history of bariatric surgery alone is not an indication for CS.

MATERNAL OBESITY AND FETAL COMPLICATIONS

In a systematic review of 39 studies and a meta-analysis of 18 studies, obese women were at increased odds of pregnancies affected by neural tube defects (NTDs), cardiovascular abnormalities, septal abnormalities, cleft lip and palate, anorectal atresia, hydrocephaly and limb reduction anomalies compared with women with a normal birth weight (BW) [21]. The risk of gastroschisis in obese women, however, was reduced. The review estimated that obesity increased the risk of an NTD by 0.47/1000 and the risk of cardiac anomaly by 0.61/1000. The investigators found no evidence that diabetes mellitus was a confounder, but could not exclude other confounding variables. It was also not possible to identify the BMI at which risk starts to increase.

Whilst the magnitude of the increased risk is small, to prevent NTDs it is recommended that all obese women should take high-dose 5 mg periconceptual folic acid supplementation and that obese women should be routinely offered an anomaly ultrasound scan [2]. However, the antenatal management is complicated by the fact that as abdominal adiposity increases, ultrasound diagnosis becomes technically more challenging. In an obese woman with a known structural anomaly, morbid obesity makes CS technically in particular more challenging and this may become a consideration in deciding the mode of delivery. In an obese woman with a known structural anomaly, morbid obesity in particular makes CS technically more challenging and this may become a consideration in deciding the mode of delivery.

The relationship between maternal obesity and the risk of stillbirth was examined in a meta-analysis which included nine studies, six with cohort and three with case–control designs [22]. The unadjusted OR of a stillbirth was 2.07 (95% CI 1.59–2.74) for obese women compared with normal women, although the mechanism to explain the association remained unclear. It is also notable that eight of the nine studies restricted their analysis to nulliparous women, three did not define stillbirth and the determination of obesity was not standardised.

Maternal obesity has been associated with aberrant intrauterine fetal growth [23]. In a systematic review and meta-analysis including 84 studies and nearly 1.1 million women, the risk of induced preterm birth was increased in overweight and obese women [relative risk (RR) 1.30; 95% CI 1.23–1.37] [24]. The risk of a low BW baby was decreased in overweight and obese women (RR 0.84; CI 0.75–0.95), but only in developing countries. The review could not adjust for confounding variables such as smoking, socioeconomic status or pre-eclampsia.

Maternal obesity has also been associated with fetal macrosomia [25]. However, the epidemiological studies were often based on self-reporting of maternal weight and were not analysed for confounding variables such as GDM or genetic influences. Furthermore, increased levels of maternal obesity have not been associated at population level with an increased incidence of fetal macrosomia or birth trauma associated with macrosomia

[26]. In a prospective study examining the relationship between BW and maternal body composition, BW was associated with maternal fat-free mass but not fat mass [26].

Not only is ultrasound estimation of fetal weight (EFW) more challenging in obese women, but the accuracy of EFW is also less if the baby is macrosomic. In the absence of GDM, therefore, the ultrasound diagnosis of a large-for-gestational age baby may mislead and potentially result in an unnecessary elective CS, or an emergency CS if an unnecessary induction of labour is unsuccessful. The adverse consequences of elective delivery based on EFW alone may escalate as the obese woman's BMI increases. It also increases the risk of repeat CS in the future which may be complicated particularly if the woman's weight has increased further.

ANAESTHETIC AND PHARMALOGICAL CONSIDERATIONS

There are important anaesthetic considerations both for labour and delivery in the obese woman, in particular, if she is morbidly obese from early pregnancy [27]. In a cohort of women who are more likely to require extra length epidural needles, the failure rate of regional anaesthesia is higher. Ultrasound may help identify structures in the vertebral column when performing the block. Intubation may be difficult in the obese woman, particularly if the neck circumference is increased, which is why regional anaesthesia is preferable to general anaesthesia. In obese women, a functioning epidural catheter should be placed in early labour (with peripheral venous access) to provide adequate analgesia and to avoid general anaesthesia in the advent of an emergency CS [27].

Maternal obesity has been associated with an increase in inpatient antenatal usage of antibiotics, analgesics and antihypertensives [28]. Obese women are also more likely to require magnesium sulphate for seizure prophylaxis in the case of pre-eclampsia or for neonatal neuroprotection in the case of preterm delivery [29]. In a study of 7799 women given magnesium, subtherapeutic levels increased as BMI increased, albeit the BMI was calculated in late pregnancy [29]. Of the obese women, 61% had subtherapeutic levels when measured at 4 hours which may be related to greater expansion of blood volume as BMI increases. To achieve therapeutic effects, it may be necessary to monitor maternal magnesium levels more frequently in obese women to minimise the risk of toxicity.

Maternal sepsis is an emerging concern in developed as well as developing countries and the early administration of broad spectrum antibiotics intravenously is considered key to minimising maternal morbidity and mortality. The measurement of maternal weight in early pregnancy is important to guide the dosing of certain antibiotics, such as gentamicin, if therapeutic levels are to be achieved in late pregnancy and peripartum due to the increased renal clearance during pregnancy.

HOSPITAL EQUIPMENT AND FACILITIES

The increase in the number of obese women attending maternity hospitals has highlighted that hospital equipment and facilities are often inadequate for the care of morbidly obese women in the delivery room, in theatre, in the emergency room and in the ward setting. An audit of each unit should be conducted to determine the availability of equipment with appropriate safe working loads and widths for the obese woman.

The audit should include the following:
- Ward and delivery beds

- Wheelchairs
- Operating tables and trolleys
- Chairs without arms
- Ultrasound scan couches
- Weighing scales
- Large BP cuffs, large specula and long amnioscopes
- Long epidural and spinal needles
- Lifting equipment
- Theatre gowns
- Toilets
- Circulation space
- Accessibility including doorway widths and thresholds

If the appropriate equipment is not available, particularly in the operating theatres and delivery suite, a procurement plan should be drawn up and implemented.

WEIGHT MANAGEMENT DURING PREGNANCY

Ideally, obese women should lose weight before they become pregnant, since obesity at the start of pregnancy is a key determinant of pregnancy outcome. However, obstetricians usually only see the woman for the first time when she presents in early pregnancy.

There is a consensus that maternal weight and height should be measured using appropriate equipment at the booking antenatal visit and the BMI calculated [1–2]. There is not a consensus, however, as to whether the woman should have her weight monitored at every antenatal visit and later in pregnancy. In the UK and Ireland, there is a concern that weighing the woman at every visit may increase maternal anxiety and that overzealous surveillance of maternal weight may distract from more important clinical issues. There is also a dearth of evidence to show that interventions during pregnancy to reduce maternal weight will succeed in improving clinical outcomes in women who are already obese.

In contrast, concerns about maternal obesity have led the Institute of Medicine in the United States of America to recommend monitoring maternal weight during pregnancy and to revise its recommendations for gestational weight gain (GWG) in 2009 [6]. The recommendations were based on the WHO BMI categories, and the recommended GWG for obese women was decreased to 5.0-9.0 kg. The committee decided that there was insufficient evidence to make specific recommendations by BMI obesity subcategories or other selective groups of women based, e.g. on ethnicity. The committee also acknowledged that there was a shortage of high quality data to base guidance on GWG and that further research is required. Despite the epidemiological associations, the relationships between maternal obesity, GWG and pregnancy outcomes are complex and the role of physical activity and dietary behaviours in modifying these relationships is incompletely understood.

By the time the obese woman presents in late pregnancy and labour, interventions to modify maternal obesity are unlikely to succeed or benefit clinically. Thus, clinicians and their multidisciplinary teams need to apply the guidelines that have been developed nationally and internationally to optimise safety for the woman and her offspring and minimise the number of cases requiring emergency interventions, particularly out-of-hours when staff resources may be low [1–3]. Efforts to prevent the development of maternal obesity may be best focused on prepregnancy and postpregnancy care [30].

Key points for clinical practice

- All women booking for antenatal care should have their weight and height measured using appropriate equipment before their BMI is calculated.
- Obese women with a mid-arm circumference >33.0 cm should have their BP measured accurately with a large cuff.
- Women who are obese should be offered a routine anomaly scan at 20-22 weeks' gestation.
- Obese women should be screened for GDM at 24-28 weeks' gestation and morbidly obese women should be screened for T2DM in early pregnancy.
- Thromboprophylaxis later in pregnancy should be based on maternal weight early in pregnancy.
- In the obese woman, labour should only be induced for clear obstetric indications and not in uncomplicated cases with a suspected big baby.
- Women with morbid obesity should be offered a consultation with an anaesthetist before delivery.
- Some antibiotic dosages may need to be adjusted therapeutically based on maternal weight.
- Women who become pregnant after bariatric surgery should be reviewed by their surgeon antenatally in case adjustment of the band is necessary.
- All maternity units should audit their equipment and facilities to make sure they are appropriate for the management and delivery of the morbidly obese woman.

REFERENCES

1. Royal College of Obstetricians and Gynaecologists (RCOG). Management of women with obesity in pregnancy, CMACE/RCOG Joint Guideline. London; RCOG, 2010.
2. Institute of Obstetricians & Gynaecologists (IOG), Royal College of Physicians of Ireland (ROPI) and Clinical Strategy and Programmes Directorate, Health Service Executive (CSPD, HSE). Obesity and pregnancy, clinical practice guideline. Dublin; IOG, ROPI, CSPD, HSE, 2011.
3. American College of Obstetricians and Gynecologists. ACOG Committee opinion no. 549: obesity in pregnancy. Obstet Gynecol 2013; 121:213–217.
4. Galliano D, Bellver J. Female obesity: short and long term consequences on the offspring. Gynecol Endocrinol 2013; 29:626–631.
5. Turner MJ. The measurement of maternal obesity: can we do better? Clin Obes 2011; 1:127–129.
6. O'Higgins AC, Doolan A, Mullaney L, et al. The relationship between gestational weight gain and fetal growth: time to take stock? J Perinatal Med 2013; 42:409–415.
7. Chu SY, Callaghan WM, Kim SY, et al. Maternal obesity and risk of gestational diabetes mellitus. Diabet Care 2007; 30:2070–2076.
8. Hogan JK, Maguire P, Farah N, et al. Body mass index and blood pressure measurement during pregnancy. Hypertens Pregnancy 2011; 30:396–400.
9. Bourjeily G, Paidas M, Khail H, et al. Pulmonary embolism in pregnancy. Lancet 2010; 375:500–512.
10. James AH, Jamison MG, Brancazio LR, et al. Venous thromboembolism during pregnancy and the postpartum period: incidence, risk factors and mortality. Am J Obstet Gynecol 2006; 194:1311–1315.
11. Jacobsen AF, Skjeldestads FE, Sandset PM. Ante- and postnatal risk factors of venous thrombosis: a hospital-based case-control study. J Thromb Haemost 2008; 6:905–912.
12. Duhl AJ, Paidas MJ, Ural SH, et al. Antithrombotic therapy and pregnancy: consensus report and recommendations for prevention and treatment of venous thromboembolism and adverse pregnancy outcomes. Am J Obstet Gynecol 2007; 197:457.e1–457.e21.
13. Lindholm ES, Altman D. Risk of obstetric anal sphincter lacerations among obese women. BJOG 2013; 120:110–115.

14. O'Dwyer V, Farah N, Fattah C, et al. The risk of caesarean section in obese women analysed by parity. Eur J Obstet Gynecol Reprod Biol 2011; 158:28–32.
15. Bujold E, Hammoud A, Schild C, et al. The role of maternal body mass index in outcomes of vaginal births after cesarean. Am J Obstet Gynecol 2005; 193:1517–1521.
16. Durnwald CP, Ehrenberg HM, Mercer BM. The impact of maternal obesity and weight gain on vaginal birth after cesarean section success. Am J Obstet Gynecol 2004; 191:954–957.
17. O'Dwyer V, O'Kelly S, Monaghan B, et al. Maternal obesity and induction of labour. Acta Obstet Gynecol Scand 2013; 92:1414–1418.
18. Bergholt T, Lim LK, Jorgensen JS, et al. Maternal body mass index in the first trimester and risk of cesarean delivery in nulliparous women in spontaneous labour. Am J Obstet Gynecol 2007; 196:163.e1-163.e5.
19. Grotegut CA, Gunatilake RP, Feng L, et al. The influence of maternal body mass index on myometrial oxytocin receptor expression in pregnancy. Reprod Sci 2013; 20:1471–1477.
20. Khan R, Dawlatly B, Chappatte O. Pregnancy outcome following bariatric surgery. Obstet Gynaecol 2013; 15:37–43.
21. Stothard KJ, Tennant PWG, Bell R, et al. Maternal overweight and obesity and the risk of congenital anomalies. JAMA 2009; 301:636–650.
22. Chu SY, Kim SY, Lau J, et al. Maternal obesity and risk of stillbirth: a metaanalysis. Am J Obstet Gynecol 2007; 197:223–228.
23. Yu CKH, Teoh TG, Robinson S. Obesity in pregnancy. BJOG 2006; 113:1117–1125.
24. McDonald SD, Han Z, Mulla S, et al. Overweight and obesity in mothers and risk of preterm birth and low birth weight infants: systematic review and meta-analysis. BMJ 2010; 34:3428.
25. Heslehurst N, Simpson H, Ells LJ, et al. The impact of maternal BMI status on pregnancy outcomes with immediate short-term obstetric resource implications: a meta-analysis. Obes Revs 2008; 9:635-683.
26. Kent E, O'Dwyer V, Fattah C, et al. Correlation between birth weight and maternal body composition. Obstet Gynecol 2013; 121:46–50.
27. Tan T, Sia AT. Anesthesia considerations in the obese gravida. Semin Perinatol 2011; 35:350–355.
28. Kennedy C, Farah N, O'Dwyer V, et al. Maternal obesity and inpatient medication usage. Clin Obes 2011; 1:147–152.
29. Tudela CM, McIntire DD, Alexander JM. Effect of maternal body mass index on serum magnesium levels given for seizure prophylaxis. Obstet Gynecol 2013; 121:314–320.
30. Turner MJ, Layte R. Obesity levels in a national cohort of women 9 months after delivery. Am J Obstet Gynecol 2013; 6:211–215.

Chapter 6

First-trimester identification of risk of pre-eclampsia

Lucy C Chappell, Shakila Thangaratinam, Jenny Myers

INTRODUCTION

Pre-eclampsia continues to be a leading cause of maternal and perinatal morbidity and mortality affecting approximately 3% of all pregnancies and 5% of healthy women in their first pregnancy [1]. The disease accounts for around 29,000 maternal deaths worldwide per year [2] and is the main cause of maternal admissions to intensive care [3]. Pre-eclampsia contributes to approximately 10% of stillbirths and 15% of preterm births [4,5], and is one of the commonest causes of iatrogenic preterm delivery accounting for occupancy of one in five neonatal intensive care costs in high-income countries [6]. The overall incidence of pre-eclampsia has remained relatively stable over the last few decades, but rates of severe pre-eclampsia have increased [7], possibly due to rising obesity in women of reproductive age.

HEALTH BURDEN OF PRE-ECLAMPSIA

Pre-eclampsia is considered to be a heterogeneous disorder with a wide spectrum of multiorgan involvement. It has been proposed that the pre-eclampsia syndrome includes several overlapping subentities of the disease including early-onset pre-eclampsia (i.e. pre-eclampsia occurring before 34 weeks' gestation) and the late-onset subtype occurring towards term [8,9]. Pre-eclampsia is now considered to comprise more than one subtype. Early-onset pre-eclampsia is associated with an increased risk of associated fetal growth restriction and stillbirth, and other adverse perinatal outcomes. As delivery is the only treatment for pre-eclampsia, early-onset disease often leads to preterm delivery of the infant once there is concern that maternal or fetal complications may occur [10]. Although the proportion of women with early-onset pre-eclampsia is less than 1% of all pregnancies, the complexity of management gives rise to large health care costs [11]. Women are often

Lucy C Chappell PhD MRCOG, Women's Health Academic Centre, King's College London, London, UK. Email: lucy.chappell@kcl.ac.uk (for correspondence)

Shakila Thangaratinam PhD MRCOG, Women's Health Research Unit, Queen Mary University of London, London, UK

Jenny Myers PhD MRCOG, Maternal and Fetal Health Research Centre, University of Manchester, Manchester, UK

admitted into a tertiary care facility and around one third experience complications, which may necessitate intensive care admission [12]. Infants born very preterm and with possible fetal growth restriction may need prolonged care for management of complications including lifelong disabilities. The additional NHS costs incurred to care for a preterm baby born before 28 weeks, and between 28 and 33 weeks, are £94,190 and £61,509, respectively [13]. A total of £939 million in extra costs for care of preterm babies per year in the NHS are linked to neonatal care such as incubation and hospital readmissions [13]. Late-onset pre-eclampsia, including pre-eclampsia at term, also poses significant health burden and accounts for the majority of the cases diagnosed with pre-eclampsia. As the underlying aetiology and pathophysiology of these phenotypes may differ, it is also plausible that one screening test at a single point in pregnancy (e.g. end of the first trimester) will not be able to identify all women at risk of all pre-eclampsia.

AETIOLOGY AND PATHOGENESIS OF PRE-ECLAMPSIA

The aetiology of pre-eclampsia is complex and not completely understood. A combination of abnormal placentation and predisposing maternal factors contribute to the development of widespread endothelial dysfunction which leads to the syndrome clinically characterised by new-onset hypertension, proteinuria and other features of multiorgan involvement (e.g. raised liver transaminases, low platelets, increased creatinine) [14]. The maternal predisposition combines immunological risk factors (first pregnancy, short duration of sperm exposure), genetic factors (increased risk if first-degree relatives affected), pre-existing vascular disease and obesity [15]. Several abnormal features of placental function and development have also been observed in pregnancies complicated by pre-eclampsia [14]. Importantly, these include studies demonstrating inadequate transformation of the maternal spiral arteries by placental trophoblast cells [16]. This can be identified clinically using uterine artery Doppler waveform analysis in the first and second trimesters [17]. It is likely that factors released by the subsequently malperfused placenta trigger the maternal endothelial dysfunction [18]. These circulating factors have been demonstrated in the maternal circulation prior to the onset of clinically detectable disease [19] and several placentally derived proteins are implicated [20].

JUSTIFICATION FOR PREDICTION

Identification of women in early pregnancy, who have a high risk of developing pre-eclampsia, alerts clinicians to the need for therapeutic prophylaxis and additional surveillance later in pregnancy. This increases the likelihood that the condition will be identified early, and potentially reducing the risk of development of complications such as severe hypertension, cerebrovascular accident, eclampsia, pulmonary oedema, renal or liver impairment, placental abruption and fetal death. Although there is currently no treatment which can prevent all cases of pre-eclampsia, there is now overwhelming evidence that low-dose aspirin [21,22] commenced in early pregnancy prevents a modest but significant number of cases, particularly early-onset pre-eclampsia, with the risk reduced by 10% for any pre-eclampsia [relative risk (RR) 0.90; 95% confidence interval (CI) 0.84–0.97] and for delivery before 34 weeks (RR 0.90; 95% CI 0.83–0.98) [21]. It is likely that prophylactic aspirin would be more acceptable to women and their healthcare professionals if they were to perceive that there is an increased risk of the disease developing. As the cost of aspirin is low, the prevention of only a small number of cases is needed to result in a substantial health economic benefit given the high cost of maternal high dependency care and neonatal intensive care.

To date, there has been no screening test that has been widely adopted into clinical practice and thus the mainstay of modern antenatal care continues to be the identification of signs of pre-eclampsia with regular measurement of blood pressure and proteinuria throughout pregnancy. Despite frequent antenatal visits, the unpredictable nature of the disease means that even close antenatal surveillance will miss a proportion of cases, especially in women with no identifiable clinical risk factors.

WHAT MAKES A GOOD PREDICTIVE TEST?

A good prediction model is one that is: accurate; validated in populations and datasets external to those used to develop the model; widely applicable in practice; acceptable to patients and ultimately improves clinical outcomes by helping clinicians and patients to make more informed decisions. This requires research studies that:

- use rigorous statistical methods to develop the model and assess accuracy;
- undertake a formal external validation (either within a further prospective study or using larger datasets gathered from other groups)
- use unambiguous definitions of predictors and reproducible measurements using methods available in clinical practice
- adjust and/or evaluate performance according to current clinical management
- involve patient groups in model development and implementation
- produce personalised risk scores that enable women and clinicians to make more informed decisions on management aspects such as commencement of aspirin early in pregnancy and the frequency of monitoring in secondary and tertiary care.

The performance of the model will naturally be limited by the strength of the predictive relationships between the measured variables and the outcome. Many of the reported studies have not fulfilled these stringent criteria, making comparisons difficult and leading to the current inability of a national body (such as the National Institute for Health and Care Excellence) to recommend any one screening test. Some authors have proposed that 'high sensitivity is a more useful attribute in early detection of pre-eclampsia than specificity because consideration of benefits, harms and costs indicates a much greater preference for minimizing false negatives than false positives, although the ideal would be to avoid both' [23].

CLINICAL RISK FACTORS FOR PREDICTION OF PRE-ECLAMPSIA

In recognition of the fact that aspirin reduces the risk of pre-eclampsia and that increased antenatal surveillance would also reduce complications of the disease, it is routine in the majority of modern high-income health care settings to assess the risk of pre-eclampsia, usually at the booking assessment at the end of the first trimester. This risk assessment has been the subject of a major research effort and the recent guidelines from the National Institute for Health and Care Excellence for management of hypertension in pregnancy [24] recommend that low-dose aspirin is commenced in those women with a baseline risk of around 10% based on clinical risk factor assessment.

The current methods for clinical assessment of pre-eclampsia risk in early pregnancy are based on maternal history [24]. However, an approach based on assessing risk through clinical history has been shown to have limited predictive accuracy, and has highlighted the need for additional tests to improve performance [25]. Recent decades have seen a plethora of studies based on biomarkers, particularly related to markers of impaired placentation, a key feature of pre-eclampsia and fetal growth restriction. There has also been considerable interest in uterine artery Doppler flow velocity waveform analysis, a noninvasive measure of uteroplacental resistance that provides an indirect estimate of abnormal placentation.

Interpretation of the varying screening tests reported depends partly on the study population. In many papers on this topic, the population studied was described as either low- or high-risk, but definitions vary between studies. Variation in study populations, combinations of biomarkers and small sample sizes have limited the ability to undertake further comparative analyses, such as meta-analyses, and have restricted the conclusions of systematic reviews. The test performance of predictive biomarkers may also depend on the definition of the outcome, such as gestation at onset of pre-eclampsia or disease of varying severity. Use of varying definitions for early- and late-onset disease and disease severity has also made direct comparisons difficult. The recent call for standardisation of pre-eclampsia research study design, incorporating minimal and optimal core datasets, standard definitions of the disease and protocols, is to be welcomed [26].

A systematic review of controlled cohort studies identified the following clinical characteristics as being associated with high risk of pre-eclampsia: previous history of pre-eclampsia (RR 7.2; 95% CI 5.9–8.8), nulliparity (2.9; 1.3–6.6), antiphospholipid antibodies (9.7; 4.3–21.8), multiple (twin) pregnancy (2.9; 2.0–4.2), family history (2.9; 1.7–4.9), raised blood pressure (diastolic ≥80 mmHg) at booking (1.4; 1.0–1.9), pre-existing diabetes (3.6; 2.5–5.0), raised body mass index (BMI) before pregnancy (2.5; 1.7–3.7) or at booking (1.6; 1.3–1.9), or maternal age ≥40 (2.0; 1.3–2.9, for multiparous women) [27]. Based on this and other work, the National Institute for Health and Care Excellence guideline identifies women with history of hypertensive disease during a previous pregnancy, chronic kidney disease, autoimmune disease such as systemic lupus erythematosus or antiphospholipid syndrome, type 1 or type 2 diabetes or chronic hypertension to be at increased risk of pre-eclampsia and requiring prophylactic treatment with aspirin [24]. In addition, the guideline recommends that women with more than one moderate risk factor (defined as nulliparity, age 40 years or older, pregnancy interval of >10 years, BMI of 35 kg/m^2 or more at booking, family history of pre-eclampsia or multiple pregnancy) are offered aspirin prophylaxis. The American College of Obstetricians and Gynecologists does not recommend routine screening to predict pre-eclampsia beyond taking an appropriate medical history to evaluate for risk factors [28]. None of the existing guidelines takes into account biomarkers or uterine Doppler for screening women for pre-eclampsia or focuses on the prediction of early-onset pre-eclampsia to improve the stratification of women at risk.

Given the important information gained from the obstetric history, recent studies [20] have therefore focused their efforts on healthy women in their first pregnancies (nulliparous), who have none of the strongest clinical risk factors for the disease. This group accounts for 50% of pre-eclampsia cases; 5% of nulliparous women are affected by pre-eclampsia and 1.3% will develop preterm disease (<37 weeks) [29]. Hence the potential benefit of an additional screening modality in nulliparous pregnancies is higher than for any other group of pregnant women.

FIRST-TRIMESTER BIOMARKERS FOR PREDICTION OF PRE-ECLAMPSIA

With developing knowledge of pre-eclampsia pathophysiology, plasma and serum biomarkers have been identified that predate its clinical presentation. The ideal biomarker would be highly sensitive and specific whilst being biologically stable, easy to measure and affordable. In practice, however, the test performance of many biomarkers is often reduced with greater time from onset of disease. The most likely scenario is development of a test that can be performed early enough to predate organ damage, but late enough to minimise false-positive and negative results. There have now been numerous studies, and many systematic reviews of such studies that have evaluated first-trimester biomarkers in pre-eclampsia. Whilst many blood biomarkers have been reported to be associated with the subsequent development of pre-eclampsia, very few have survived external validation. Those which consistently show some potential include placenta growth factor (PlGF), pregnancy associated plasma protein-A (PAPP-A), placental protein-13 (PP-13) and disintegrin and metalloproteinase domain-containing protein 12 (ADAM-12). The relative contribution of each biomarker to prediction algorithms has varied across studies and is dependent on the population studied (e.g. the presence of comorbidity), the timing of the measurement and the pre-eclampsia phenotype chosen as the endpoint. Several studies have included individual biomarkers within prediction models despite measurement in only a small proportion of the study population [30]; very few of the biomarkers have been validated in independent cohorts, an essential step prior to widespread adoption into clinical practice.

A number of large studies have correlated decreased maternal PlGF concentrations with the development of pre-eclampsia later in pregnancy. A recent systematic review of 15 predictive studies of angiogenic factors reported a summary diagnostic odds ratio of 9.0 (95% CI 5.6–14.5), corresponding to both sensitivities and specificities of 0.75, or a sensitivity of 0.32 for a 5% false-positive rate [31]. However, this systematic review included studies testing up to 30 weeks of gestation; future meta-analyses need to report the screening performance stratified by gestation, with PlGF in isolation and in combination. A comprehensive list of studies reporting PlGF and other angiogenic markers is given in a recent review [32].

Similar significant associations have been detected for PP13 [33], PAPP-A and ADAM-12 [34] in preliminary studies and there has also been interest in biochemical markers used in clinical practice for Down's syndrome screening such as PAPP-A, human chorionic gonadotrophin (hCG) and serum alpha-feto protein (AFP), but few have sufficient sensitivity for routine clinical adaptation, or have been externally validated [35]. The limited test performance of biomarkers in isolation has led several research groups to propose combining markers, with or without the addition of uterine artery Doppler or clinical characteristics.

FIRST-TRIMESTER UTERINE ARTERY DOPPLER FOR PREDICTION OF PRE-ECLAMPSIA

A recent systematic review (1951–2012) identified 18 studies (55,974 women) evaluating the accuracy of first-trimester Doppler in predicting pre-eclampsia [17]. The sensitivity and specificity of abnormal flow velocity waveform for early-onset pre-eclampsia were 0.48 (95% CI 0.39–0.57) and 0.92 (95% CI 0.89–0.95) respectively. The sensitivity and specificity for predicting any pre-eclampsia were 0.26 (95% CI 0.23–0.31) and 0.15 (95% CI 0.12–0.19), respectively. The findings of this review highlight the need for development of prediction models, incorporating the clinical characteristics with uterine artery Doppler to increase the accuracy of risk assessment.

Given the disappointing results of screening tests in isolation, studies have combined biomarker measurement with uterine artery Doppler results with varying success. A large prospective cohort study (7797 women) combined first-trimester uterine artery Doppler, PAPP-A and PlGF in conjunction with mean arterial pressure and clinical characteristics (ethnicity, previous/family history of pre-eclampsia and parity). It reported respective test sensitivities and specificities of 0.93 and 0.95, respectively, for early-onset pre-eclampsia and 0.35 and 0.95, respectively, for late-onset disease [36]. A further large case–control study from this group evaluated a similar combination of clinical and biochemical parameters and uterine artery Dopplers [15]. However, in several of these and similar studies, algorithms have been developed using data from women with very different pretest probabilities. Several have combined healthy nulliparous (5% risk) and multiparous women (<0.3% risk) with those with known risk factors (previous pre-eclampsia, concurrent medical disease, 20% risk). These algorithms will, by definition, overperform in women with the highest pretest probability and underperform in those who would most benefit from the test (healthy nulliparous women). It follows that if these algorithms were introduced in their current format, the detection rate in first pregnancies would be low with a large proportion of cases missed. In order for prediction to be improved for healthy nulliparous women, algorithms need to be designed specifically for this group.

The performance of multivariate models is also dependent on the prevalence of the disease. A recent study which combined biochemical and clinical risk factors demonstrated very poor performance for the detection of pre-eclampsia, although this study did not include uterine artery Doppler [37].

A comprehensive systematic review of 144 studies assessed the accuracy of 27 tests in the prediction of pre-eclampsia [38]. Most of these studies were limited by their poor quality and potential threats to validity (through lack of blinding, poor reporting of test description and inadequate reference standard). Many studies did not provide separate risk-specific results, but included pregnant women across the clinical risk spectrum. The tests with high specificity had low sensitivity. The main recommendation from this work (commissioned by the Health Technology Assessment programme and reported in 2008) was not to offer testing, in view of the poor predictive accuracy, but to perform robust evaluation of new tests or those with reported high levels of both sensitivity and specificity in the clinical setting where they will be applied. Future studies should investigate combinations of markers, and evaluate the added value of new tests to the risk profile based on the clinical history. More importantly, the report recommended that predictive models developed in the future should be validated using individual patient data diagnostic meta-analysis. This is a method in which individual patient data from original studies are obtained directly from the researchers and re-analysed centrally in combination with data from other studies, rather than pooling summary information from each study. This type of 'individual patient data' meta-analysis takes longer and requires specific expertise, but is considered to provide more reliable results than pooling aggregate data (as in a conventional meta-analysis).

RECOMMENDATIONS FOR CLINICAL PRACTICE

By far the strongest risk factor for the development of pre-eclampsia is the occurrence of the condition in a previous pregnancy. The recurrence of the disease varies from 10% to 50% depending on the gestation at onset and severity of the disease [39]. It is therefore now routine practice to commence aspirin in women previously affected and to instigate a programme of closer antenatal surveillance. At present there is no biomarker test which reliably improves or excludes risk assessment for pre-eclampsia and/or fetal growth restriction in women with a previous history of the disease [30] and there is therefore no added benefit of a biochemical/ biophysical test in the care of this group of women. This also applies to women who have underlying medical disease such as hypertension, diabetes or other autoimmune conditions, as these women will also justify the prescription of aspirin and intense antenatal surveillance based on a significantly elevated risk (17–20%) of developing pre-eclampsia [40,41]. Conversely, women in their second and subsequent pregnancies with previous uncomplicated pregnancies have a very low incidence of the disease (<0.3%) [15], although this may be increased by a long inter-pregnancy interval or a new partner. In the absence of any other medical risk factors, the pretest probability of the condition developing in these women is very low and extremely unlikely to be altered substantially by additional screening.

On the basis of current evidence, the detection rate for preterm pre-eclampsia (<37 weeks), using established risk factors and biochemical variables measured in the first trimester, is likely to be 55–70% in low risk nulliparous women. Detection rates for later onset disease will, however, be considerably lower [42]. First-trimester screening alone is therefore highly unlikely to meet the robust demands of a 'catch all' predictive test for the disease. This likely reflects the longer temporal relationship between the test being performed and the disease developing, but also the heterogeneous nature of the condition. Recognition of term pre-eclampsia remains important as approximately two thirds of cases present after 37 weeks' gestation and severe maternal morbidity and mortality are common in this group [43]. Enthusiasm is therefore mounting for introduction of a third-trimester screening to improve the detection of later onset disease, as recently reported. These studies provide new evidence to suggest that additional cases of late preterm and early term disease can be detected in the third trimester by measurement of angiogenic factors, particularly PlGF. Whilst there are modest cost implications to an additional screening time point, this important development in pre-eclampsia screening now requires prospective evaluation. Enhanced detection of cases in the third trimester would translate to a significant reduction in the burden of disease by early identification of cases, appropriate surveillance and intervention (e.g. antenatal steroids) and optimal timing of delivery with the intention of reducing the frequency of severe complications [44].

RECOMMENDATIONS FOR RESEARCH

The lack of externally validated screening tests for pre-eclampsia has led to two recent commissioned calls for research from the National Institute for Health Research (NIHR). Recognising that recent systematic reviews have failed to identify any individual marker or combination of markers for this purpose, the Health Technology Assessment Programme of the NIHR has recently invited research consortia to address the following research question through a new evidence synthesis, to include recent studies of both novel and previously used biomarkers: 'Is there any evidence that in the first or second trimester of pregnancy any biomarkers, combinations of biomarkers or risk models are useful for predicting the subsequent onset of pre-eclampsia? Would any be suitable for screening women?' Given the lack of a clinically applicable screening test despite the numerous systematic reviews on the topic, a new approach, such as an individual patient data meta-analysis, is now required to address this in order to yield a meaningful answer. At the same time as this evidence synthesis, the Efficacy and Mechanism Evaluation Programme has commissioned a parallel piece of research 'for studies of novel biochemical markers, ultrasound techniques, combinations of markers or risk models or other prognostic markers which can be used early in pregnancy to predict the risk of pre-eclampsia later in the pregnancy'. It is expected that the successful research groups who obtain funding will report results in the next 2–4 years.

CONCLUSION

Pre-eclampsia is a common and important complication of pregnancy. There is a need for an accurate predictive test for pre-eclampsia, with a screening strategy that may need to encompass different time points in pregnancy to enable prediction of the varying phenotypes of the disease. Pregnant women at increased risk of pre-eclampsia should be monitored closely and commenced on prophylactic interventions such as aspirin in order to reduce adverse outcomes. Stratification of care with increased surveillance for those at greater risk and reassurance and reduced surveillance for women at low risk may be beneficial to a substantial proportion of the screened population. Early commencement of prophylactic interventions has the potential for maximal benefit [22]. A clinically applicable screening test is likely to include markers of abnormal placentation and of preclinical maternal features of the disease. The most convincing evidence for predicting future pre-eclampsia lies in combined screening techniques. A combination of clinical characteristics and biomarker analysis may offer the best test performance, and future research should be focused in this direction, with appropriate external validation prior to widespread uptake. There is little doubt that as our screening strategy improves, greater mechanistic understanding will follow enabling novel targeted prophylactic interventions to be developed with the aim of ameliorating the major impact of pre-eclampsia on the lives of mothers and babies.

Key points for clinical practice

- Pre-eclampsia appears to include several overlapping subentities including early- and late-onset disease; as the underlying aetiology and pathophysiology of these phenotypes may differ, one screening test (in the first trimester) may not be able to identify all women at risk of pre-eclampsia.
- Guidelines from the UK National Institute for Health and Care Excellence recommend assessment of pre-eclampsia risk based on clinical history, with commencement of low-dose aspirin in those with a baseline risk of around 10%.
- First trimester biomarkers including placenta growth factor (PlGF) and pregnancy-associated plasma protein-A (PAPP-A) have been reported to be associated with the subsequent

development of pre-eclampsia, but no biomarker has yet been validated and recommended for routine use in clinical practice.

- Other studies have combined biomarker measurement with first trimester uterine artery Doppler results with varying success, but no combination is yet in routine clinical practice.

- Previous history of pre-eclampsia or chronic medical conditions (such as hypertension or diabetes) increase the risk of pre-eclampsia and low-dose prophylactic aspirin is recommended.

- For other women, including nulliparous women without clear risk factors, there is no recommended biomarker or Doppler-based screening test.

- Future research is needed to elucidate the optimal timing and modality of screening for pre-eclampsia, with the aim of enabling prediction and subsequent prevention of the disease.

REFERENCES

1. Steegers EA, von Dadelszen P, Duvekot JJ, et al. Lancet 2010; 376:631–644.
2. Kassebaum NJ, Bertozzi-Villa A, Coggeshall MS, et al. Global, regional, and national levels and causes of maternal mortality during 1990-2013: a systematic analysis for the Global Burden of Disease Study 2013. Lancet 2014; 384:980–1004.
3. Tang LC, Kwok AC, Wong AY, et al. Critical care in obstetrical patients: an eight-year review. Chin Med J (Engl) 1997; 110:936–941.
4. Gardosi J, Kady SM, McGeown P, et al. Classification of stillbirth by relevant condition at death (ReCoDe): population-based cohort study. BMJ 2005; 331:1113–1117.
5. Iams JD, Goldenberg RL, Mercer BM, et al. The preterm prediction study: recurrence risk of spontaneous preterm birth. National Institute of Child Health and Human Development Maternal-Fetal Medicine Units Network. Am J Obstet Gynecol 1998; 178:1035–1040.
6. Sibai BM. Preeclampsia as a cause of preterm and late preterm (near-term) births. Semin Perinatol 2006; 30:16–19.
7. Ananth CV, Keyes KM, Wapner RJ. Pre-eclampsia rates in the United States, 1980-2010: age-period-cohort analysis. BMJ 2013; 347:f6564.
8. Crispi F, Dominguez C, Llurba E, et al. Placental angiogenic growth factors and uterine artery Doppler findings for characterization of different subsets in preeclampsia and in isolated intrauterine growth restriction. Am J Obstet Gynecol 2006; 195:201–207.
9. Valensise H, Vasapollo B, Gagliardi G, et al. Early and late preeclampsia: two different maternal hemodynamic states in the latent phase of the disease. Hypertension 2008; 52:873–880.
10. Lisonkova S, Joseph KS. Incidence of preeclampsia: risk factors and outcomes associated with early- versus late-onset disease. Am J Obstet Gynecol 2013; 209:544.e1–544.e12.
11. Murphy DJ, Stirrat GM. Mortality and morbidity associated with early-onset preeclampsia. Hyperten Pregnancy 2000; 19:221–231.
12. Churchill D, Duley L, Thornton JG, et al. Interventionist versus expectant care for severe pre-eclampsia between 24 and 34 weeks' gestation. Cochrane Database Syst Rev 2013; 7:CD003106.
13. Mangham LJ, Petrou S, Doyle LW, et al. The cost of preterm birth throughout childhood in England and Wales. Pediatrics 2009; 123:e312–e327.
14. Redman CW, Sargent IL, Staff AC. IFPA Senior Award Lecture: making sense of pre-eclampsia––two placental causes of preeclampsia? Placenta 2014; 35 Suppl:S20–S25.
15. Akolekar R, Syngelaki A, Sarquis R, et al. Prediction of early, intermediate and late pre-eclampsia from maternal factors, biophysical and biochemical markers at 11–13 weeks. Prenat Diagn 2011; 31:66–74.
16. Pijnenborg R, Vercruysse L, Verbist L, et al. Interaction of interstitial trophoblast with placental bed capillaries and venules of normotensive and pre-eclamptic pregnancies. Placenta 1998; 19:569–575.
17. Velauthar L, Plana MN, Kalidindi M, et al. First-trimester uterine artery Doppler and adverse pregnancy outcome: a meta-analysis involving 55,974 women. Ultrasound Obstet Gynecol 2014; 43:500–507.
18. Roberts JM, Lain KY. Recent insights into the pathogenesis of pre-eclampsia. Placenta 2002; 23:359–372.
19. Myers J, Mires G, Macleod M, et al. In preeclampsia, the circulating factors capable of altering in vitro endothelial function precede clinical disease. Hypertension 2005; 45:258–263.

20. Myers JE, Kenny LC, McCowan LM, et al. Angiogenic factors combined with clinical risk factors to predict preterm pre-eclampsia in nulliparous women: a predictive test accuracy study. BJOG 2013; 120:1215–1223.
21. Askie LM, Duley L, Henderson-Smart DJ, et al. Antiplatelet agents for prevention of pre-eclampsia: a meta-analysis of individual patient data. Lancet 2007; 369:1791–1798.
22. Bujold E, Roberge S, Lacasse Y, et al. Prevention of preeclampsia and intrauterine growth restriction with aspirin started in early pregnancy: a meta-analysis. Obstet Gynecol 2010; 116:402–414.
23. Cnossen JS, ter Riet G, Mol BW, et al. Are tests for predicting pre-eclampsia good enough to make screening viable? A review of reviews and critical appraisal. Acta Obstet Gynecol Scand 2009; 88:758–765.
24. National Institute for Health and Care Excellence (NICE). Hypertension in pregnancy: the management of hypertensive disorders during pregnancy, CG107. London; NICE, 2010.
25. Giguere Y, Charland M, Bujold E, et al. Combining biochemical and ultrasonographic markers in predicting preeclampsia: a systematic review. Clin Chem 2010; 56:361–375.
26. Myatt L, Redman CW, Staff AC, et al. Strategy for standardization of preeclampsia research study design. Hypertension 2014; 63:1293–1301.
27. Duckitt K, Harrington D. Risk factors for pre-eclampsia at antenatal booking: systematic review of controlled studies. BMJ 2005; 330:565.
28. American College of Obstetricians and Gynecologists, Task Force on Hypertension in Pregnancy. Hypertension in pregnancy. Report of the American College of Obstetricians and Gynecologists' Task Force on Hypertension in Pregnancy. Obstet Gynecol 2013; 122:1122–1131.
29. North RA, McCowan LM, Dekker GA, et al. Clinical risk prediction for pre-eclampsia in nulliparous women: development of model in international prospective cohort. BMJ 2011; 342:d1875.
30. Akolekar R, Syngelaki A, Poon L, et al. Competing risks model in early screening for preeclampsia by biophysical and biochemical markers. Fetal Diagn Ther 2013; 33:8–15.
31. Kleinrouweler CE, Wiegerinck MM, Ris-Stalpers C, et al. Accuracy of circulating placental growth factor, vascular endothelial growth factor, soluble fms-like tyrosine kinase 1 and soluble endoglin in the prediction of pre-eclampsia: a systematic review and meta-analysis. BJOG 2012; 119:778–787.
32. Andraweera PH, Dekker GA, Roberts CT. The vascular endothelial growth factor family in adverse pregnancy outcomes. Hum Reprod Update 2012; 18:436–457.
33. Odibo AO, Zhong Y, Goetzinger KR, et al. First-trimester placental protein 13, PAPP-A, uterine artery Doppler and maternal characteristics in the prediction of pre-eclampsia. Placenta 2011; 32:598–602.
34. Odibo AO, Patel KR, Spitalnik A, et al. Placental pathology, first-trimester biomarkers and adverse pregnancy outcomes. J Perinatol 2014; 34:186–191.
35. Morris RK, Cnossen JS, Langejans M, et al. Serum screening with Down's syndrome markers to predict pre-eclampsia and small for gestational age: systematic review and meta-analysis. BMC Pregnancy Childbirth 2008; 8:33.
36. Poon LC, Kametas NA, Maiz N, et al. First-trimester prediction of hypertensive disorders in pregnancy. Hypertension 2009; 53:812–818.
37. Giguere Y, Masse J, Theriault S, et al. Screening for pre-eclampsia early in pregnancy: performance of a multivariable model combining clinical characteristics and biochemical markers. BJOG 2015; 122:402–410.
38. Meads CA, Cnossen JS, Meher S, et al. Methods of prediction and prevention of pre-eclampsia: systematic reviews of accuracy and effectiveness literature with economic modelling. Health Technol Assess 2008; 12:iii-iv, 1–270.
39. Dildy GA 3rd, Belfort MA, Smulian JC. Preeclampsia recurrence and prevention. Semin Perinatol 2007; 31:135–141.
40. Chappell LC, Enye S, Seed P, et al. Adverse perinatal outcomes and risk factors for preeclampsia in women with chronic hypertension: a prospective study. Hypertension 2008; 51:1002–1009.
41. McCance DR, Holmes VA, Maresh MJ, et al. Vitamins C and E for prevention of pre-eclampsia in women with type 1 diabetes (DAPIT): a randomised placebo-controlled trial. Lancet 2010; 376:259–266.
42. Myatt L, Clifton RG, Roberts JM, et al. First-trimester prediction of preeclampsia in nulliparous women at low risk. Obstet Gynecol 2012; 119:1234–1242.
43. Smith GC. Researching new methods of screening for adverse pregnancy outcome: lessons from pre-eclampsia. PLoS Med 2012; 9:e1001274.
44. Koopmans CM, Bijlenga D, Groen H, et al. Induction of labour versus expectant monitoring for gestational hypertension or mild pre-eclampsia after 36 weeks' gestation (HYPITAT): a multicentre, open-label randomised controlled trial. Lancet 2009; 374:979–988.

Chapter 7

Selective progesterone receptor modulators in gynaecology

Vikram Sinai Talaulikar, Isaac Manyonda

INTRODUCTION

Progesterone is an endogenous steroid hormone that plays a critical role in human reproductive physiology. It belongs to a group of steroid hormones called the progestogens, and is a crucial metabolic intermediate in the production of sex hormones and the corticosteroids. Its physiological effects impact the processes of endometrial differentiation in the menstrual cycle (decidualisation), ovulation, embryo implantation and successful development of pregnancy. During pregnancy, progesterone secretion is associated with quiescence of the myometrium, and a decrease in its concentration may be one of the signals associated with the onset of labour. It is also important for the development of the mammary gland and exerts biologic effects on a range of organ systems including cardiovascular, central nervous system and bone. The effects of progesterone on target tissues are mediated via the progesterone receptor (PR) that belongs to the nuclear receptor family [1]. The PR exists as three separate isoforms (A, B and C) expressed from a single gene. The PR functions as a ligand-activated transcription factor to regulate the expression of specific sets of target genes.

The first PR antagonist to be identified was RU-486 (mifepristone) discovered in 1980. Since then, a number of synthetic PR ligands with mixed activity have been discovered which act as agonists and/or antagonists in a tissue-specific manner, and are termed the selective PR modulators (SPRMs). The PR ligands can possess activity ranging from pure agonist activity through mixed agonist/antagonist activity to pure antagonist activity. It is generally believed that the tissue ratio of PR-A/PR-B receptors is crucial for the SPRM effect.

In this chapter, the term SPRM will be used to describe all PR ligands that show some degree of PR receptor agonistic and antagonistic activity. These compounds have a huge potential for use in the treatment of a range of conditions of the female reproductive system including use as contraceptives, the prevention of pregnancy loss and preterm labour, the alleviation of dysfunctional uterine bleeding (DUB), the treatment of endometriosis and most recently and promising, the treatment of uterine fibroids.

Vikram Sinai Talaulikar MD MRCOG, Reproductive Medicine Unit, University College London Hospital, London, UK

Isaac Manyonda PhD MRCOG, Department of Obstetrics and Gynaecology, St George's Hospital and University of London, London, UK. Email: imanyond@sgul.ac.uk (for correspondence)

Immediate examples of SPRMs that have been the subject of recent clinical trials or research studies in relation to the treatment of gynaecological conditions include RU-486 (mifepristone), CDB-4124 (telapristone), CP-8947 and J-867 (asoprisnil) and CDB-2914 [ulipristal acetate (UA)].

MECHANISMS OF ACTION OF SPRMS

Contraception

Since progesterone is critical for ovulation, successful embryo implantation and maintenance of early pregnancy, SPRMs are the obvious candidates for potential clinical utility in these areas. Daily doses of mifepristone (2–5 mg), telapristone (12.5–50 mg) and ulipristal (5–10 mg) inhibit ovulation in normal women [2–6], but asoprisnil, in contrast, is not as effective in inhibiting ovulation [7,8]. The amenorrhoea that occurs with SPRMs is associated with serum levels of oestradiol equivalent to those seen in the early follicular phase of the normal menstrual cycle [8]. Amongst all SPRMs, mifepristone has unique antagonist activities and it is the only one that has been used for medical termination of pregnancy. Some in vitro studies have suggested that mifepristone may inhibit endometrial receptivity [15] and tubal contractility [16] and that UA may inhibit human sperm hyperactivation [17], as well as ciliary beating and muscular contraction in the human fallopian tube [18].

Mifepristone, one of the earliest progesterone antagonists on the market, has been commonly used for first trimester medical termination of pregnancy with or without misoprostol. It is also used in the management of second trimester medical termination of pregnancy and intrauterine fetal death (IUFD) in conjunction with misoprostol. It is a selective antagonist of the PR at low doses and blocks the glucocorticoid receptor at higher doses [19]. For purposes of pregnancy termination, it is used in doses of 200–800 mg and its efficacy is well proven. A Cochrane review compared three regimens for the medical termination of first trimester pregnancy [20]. Fifty-eight trials were included in the review. In the combined regimen (mifepristone/prostaglandin), a mifepristone dose of 200 mg showed similar efficacy to a dose of 600 mg in achieving complete abortion [four trials, relative risk (RR) 1.07; 95% confidence interval (CI) 0.87–1.32]. Mifepristone on its own was less effective when compared to the combined regimen mifepristone/prostaglandin (RR 3.76; 95% CI 2.30–6.15). Five trials compared prostaglandin alone to the combined regimen (mifepristone/prostaglandin). All but one reported higher effectiveness with the combined regimen. The authors concluded that in the combined regimen, the dose of mifepristone could be lowered to 200 mg without significantly decreasing the method's effectiveness [20].

One study compared different methods of second trimester medical terminationof pregnancy for their efficacy and side effects [21]. Forty randomised controlled trials (RCTs) were included addressing various agents for pregnancy termination and methodsof administration. Medical abortion in the second trimester using the combination of mifepristone and misoprostol appeared to have the highest efficacy and shortest abortion time interval. Although misoprostol on its own was an effective inductive agent, it was more effective when combined with mifepristone [21].

CLINICAL UTILITY OF SPRMS FOR THE MANAGEMENT OF GYNAECOLOGICAL CONDITIONS

Uterine fibroids

Whilst it has long been known that oestrogen promotes fibroid growth, biochemical and clinical studies have suggested that progesterone and PR can also enhance proliferative activity in fibroids [2,9]. These early observations raised the possibility that SPRMs could be useful in the medical management of uterine fibroids. Progesterone has dual actions on fibroid growth. It stimulates growth by upregulating endothelial growth factor and Bcl-2 and downregulating tumour necrosis factor-α expression whilst it inhibits growth by downregulating insulin like growth factor-I (IGF-I) expression [2,9]. Fibroid cells demonstrate higher concentrations of oestrogen receptors, and equally higher expression of mRNA and differential expression of PRs compared to surrounding myometrium. These differences account for the differential action of SPRMs on fibroids as compared to normal myometrium.

Several studies have suggested at least six pathways by which SPRMs can affect fibroids:

1. UA downregulates the expression of angiogenic growth factors such as vascular endothelial growth factor and their receptors in cultured fibroid cells [10]. This may result in the suppression of neovascularisation, cell proliferation and survival [2].
2. UA and asoprisnil inhibit the proliferation of cultured fibroid cells and induce apoptosis by upregulating cleaved caspase 3 and downregulating Bcl-2 [2,10,11].
3. UA also increases the expression of matrix metalloproteinases and decreases the expression of tissue inhibitor of metalloproteinases and collagens in cultured fibroid cells. This may reduce collagen deposition in the extracellular spaces of fibroids, impairing tissue integrity [2,10,12]. Asoprisnil downregulates collagen synthesis in cultured human uterine leiomyoma cells through upregulating extracellular matrix metalloproteinase inducer [13].
4. Asoprisnil and UA have been shown to modulate the ratio of PR isoforms (PR-A and PR-B) in the cultured leiomyoma cells [14]. They decreased the cell viability; suppressed the expression of growth factors, angiogenic factors and their receptors in those cells; and induced apoptosis through activating the mitochondrial and tumour necrosis factor-related apoptosis-inducing ligand (TRAIL) pathways and eliciting endoplasmic reticulum stress. Furthermore, these compounds suppressed types I and III collagen synthesis by modulating extracellular matrix remodelling enzymes in cultured leiomyoma cells without affecting those syntheses in cultured normal myometrial cells [14,8].
5. Mifepristone and asoprisnil have also been associated with a decrease in the uterine artery blood flow [8].

Management of intrauterine fetal death

In cases of late IUFD, induction of labour in a woman with an unscarred uterus is recommended using a combination of mifepristone and a prostaglandin preparation (first-line intervention) [22]. In a case series of 96 women with a late fetal death, the combination of mifepristone and misoprostol gave an average duration of labour of 8 hours. The addition of mifepristone appeared to reduce the time interval by about 7 hours compared with published regimens not including mifepristone, but there was no other apparent benefit [23]. A single 200 mg dose of mifepristone is appropriate for this indication [22].

For induction of labour in a woman with prior lower segment caesarean section with IUFD, a discussion of the safety and benefits of induction of labour should be undertaken with a consultant obstetrician, and mifepristone can be used alone to increase the chance of labour significantly within 72 hours (avoiding the use of prostaglandin) [22]. An RCT of oral mifepristone alone (200 mg three times a day for 2 days) was compared with placebo in women with an IUFD. Labour occurred within 72 hours in significantly more women in the mifepristone group (63% vs. 17%, $P < 0.001$) [22,24]. Use of mifepristone in this context is off-label [25]. Mifepristone 600 mg once daily for 2 days can also be used [22,25].

Emergency contraception

Both mifepristone and UA have been used for emergency contraception. Early studies used mifepristone at a dose of 600 mg within 72 hours of unprotected sexual intercourse. A subsequent study by the World Health Organization (WHO) confirmed that lower doses of mifepristone (50 and 10 mg) were equally effective [26]. A Cochrane review was conducted to determine which emergency contraception method following unprotected intercourse is the most effective, safe and convenient to prevent pregnancy [27]. One hundred trials with 55,666 women were included. Most trials were conducted in China (86%). Meta-analysis indicated that mid-dose mifepristone (25–50 mg) (20 trials; RR 0.64; 95% CI 0.45–0.92) or low-dose mifepristone (<25 mg) (11 trials; RR 0.70; 95% CI 0.50–0.97) was significantly more effective than levonorgestrel (LNG), but the difference was marginal when only high-quality studies were included (four trials; RR 0.70; 95% CI 0.49–1.01). Low-dose mifepristone was less effective than mid-dose mifepristone (25 trials; RR 0.73; 95% CI 0.55–0.97). This difference was not statistically significant when only high-quality trials were considered (six trials; RR 0.75; 95% CI 0.50–1.10). The RR of effectiveness between the groups using UA and LNG within 72 hours of unprotected sexual intercourse was 0.63 (95% CI 0.37–1.07). It was not evident that the coitus-to-treatment time affected the effectiveness of mifepristone and uliprital [27]. Mifepristone (all doses) (three trials; RR 0.14; 95% CI 0.05–0.41) and LNG (five trials; RR 0.54; 95% CI 0.36–0.80) were more effective than the Yuzpe regimen in preventing pregnancy. As a side effect of administration of emergency contraceptive, antiprogestogen methods caused changes in subsequent menses [27]. UA users were more likely to have a menstrual return after the expected date. Menstrual delay was also the main adverse effect of mifepristone and seemed to be dose related. The authors concluded that intermediate-dose mifepristone (25–50 mg) was superior to LNG and Yuzpe regimens [27].

The apparently superior efficacy of mifepristone over LNG may arise from its additional postovulatory mechanism of action in inhibiting endometrial receptivity and tubal contractility. Since 2009, the oral tablet containing 30 mg UA has been marketed as a single dose emergency contraceptive to be taken within 120 hours of unprotected sexual intercourse. UA was shown in two large RCTs to be as effective as LNG for emergency contraception when administered within 72 hours of unprotected sexual intercourse [28,29]. The second study also included 100 subjects taking UA between 72 and 120 hours after unprotected intercourse in which no pregnancy was observed. The main mechanism of action of UA in this situation is to delay or inhibit ovulation, and such an effect remains evident even after the onset but before the peak of the luteinising hormone surge [30–32].

It has also been postulated that UA may alter endometrial receptivity, exerting an anti-implantation effect, as well as altering tubal and sperm functions [32].

Endometriosis and dysfunctional uterine bleeding

A small number of clinical studies have demonstrated a potential role for SPRMs in the treatment of endometriosis. Mifepristone administered at a dose of 50 mg daily has been shown to reduce pain and induce regression of endometriosis [19,33]. Asoprisnil and telapristone have also been reported to relieve pain associated with endometriosis [2,19,34,35]. When used for the treatment of endometriosis, SPRMs may exert their effects by a direct effect on the endometrial deposits. However, more studies on both their efficacy and long-term effects on endometrium are needed before they can be used in clinical practice for the treatment of endometriosis.

The use of SPRMs for DUB also needs further work. The observation of suppression of bleeding in women with uterine fibroids treated with SPRMs and improvement in breakthrough bleeding on progestin treatment following SPRM administration point towards likely benefit of SPRMs in DUB [19,36,37].

Uterine fibroids

Mifepristone (RU-486) was initially used for the treatment of fibroids in doses ranging from 12.5 to 50 mg daily and the study group reported a reduction in uterine/fibroid volume of 40–50%, with amenorrhoea in most subjects [38]. This report was corroborated by a paper a year later from a group who used RU-486 at a dose of 5 or 10 mg per day for 1 year, and found that it was effective in decreasing mean uterine volume by 50%, whilst amenorrhoea occurred in 40–70% of the subjects [39]. Adverse effects included vasomotor symptoms, but no change in bone mineral density was noted. Hot flushes were increased over baseline in the 10 mg group, but 5 mg per day did not increase the incidence of vasomotor symptoms. Simple hyperplasia was noted in 28% of the women. This study therefore suggested that a dose as low as 5 mg per day of mifepristone could be efficacious for the treatment of uterine fibroids, with few side effects [39]. This study was followed by an RCT, but this was a small study which included 42 women in a double-blind placebo-controlled study design over a period of 6 months [40]. The authors reported significant improvements in quality of life and significant reduction in anaemia rates and uterine volume. Moreover, women were more likely to become amenorrhoeic if they were treated with a low dose of mifepristone. In a larger randomised trial, 100 women were assigned to mifepristone 5 or 10 mg daily for 3 months without a placebo group. With both doses, there were equivalent reductions in fibroid and uterine volumes and symptomatic improvements [41].

Telapristone (CDB-4124)

A clinical trial (phase I/II) evaluated the efficacy of CDB-4124 in symptomatic fibroids. This small 3-month study comprising 30 women compared oral doses of 12.5, 25 and 50 mg with the gonadotropin-releasing hormone (GnRH) analogue Lupron and a placebo [42]. There was a significant reduction in tumour size and amount of bleeding with telapristone treatment.

One study examined the endometrial histology in 58 premenopausal women treated with telapristone for endometriosis or fibroids in two clinical trials [43]. Endometrial biopsies obtained after 3 or 6 months with doses of 12.5, 25 or 50 mg daily oral CDB-4124 were reviewed independently by three pathologists. Consensus diagnoses using the WHO hyperplasia scoring system, comments on specific histological features and clinical annotation were collected and analysed. The majority of the endometrial biopsies (103 of 174 biopsies) contained histological changes that are not seen during normal menstrual cycles. The histology of telapristone-treated patients was generally inactive or atrophic, and less frequently, proliferative or secretory, superimposed upon which were novel changes including formation of cystically dilated glands, and secretory changes co-existing with mitoses and apoptotic bodies. Cystic glands in the telapristone-treated subjects correlated with increased endometrial thickness observed by ultrasound. None of the telapristone-treated patients developed endometrial carcinoma or hyperplasia whilst on therapy [43].

Asoprisnil (J-867)

It has high tissue selectivity and binds to PRs with a threefold greater binding affinity than progesterone [44]. The initial phase I studies established that asoprisnil induced a reversible suppression of menstruation, whilst having variable effects on ovulation [7]. The phase II multicentre double-blind placebo-controlled studies by the same group of researchers compared the efficacy and safety of three doses (5, 10 and 25 mg and placebo) in 129 women over 12 weeks [45,46]. Asoprisnil reduced the uterine and fibroid volumes in a dose-dependent manner. There was a dose-dependent decrease in menorrhagia scores in women with menorrhagia at baseline, whilst amenorrhoea rates increased as the dose increased (28.1% with 5 mg, 64.3% with 10 mg and 83.3% with 25 mg), but with no increase in the rates of unscheduled bleeding in all three asoprisnil groups. Bloating was significantly reduced in the 10 and 25 mg groups, and pelvic pressure significantly reduced in the 25 mg group. Compared to placebo, haemoglobin levels were improved in all three treatment groups, whilst adverse effects were evenly distributed.

UA (CDB-2914)

From 2012, UA has been used for the preoperative treatment of moderate-to-severe symptoms of uterine fibroids in adult women of reproductive age (one 5 mg tablet per day for up to 3 months--the 3-month course can be repeated once). It exerts proapoptotic antiproliferative effects on fibroid cells without suppressing oestrogen to nonphysiologic levels. In the first trial in which UA was given at 10 or 20 mg in comparison against placebo for three cycles, UA showed a 92% reduction in bleeding versus 19% with placebo. Leiomyoma volume was significantly reduced with ulipristal administration (placebo 6%; CDB-2914, -29%; $P = 0.01$) [47]. UA eliminated menstrual bleeding and inhibited ovulation (% ovulatory cycles: CDB-2914, 20%; PLC 83%; $P = 0.001$). CDB-2914 improved the concern scores of the uterine leiomyoma symptom quality-of-life subscale ($P = 0.04$). One woman given ulipristal developed endometrial cystic hyperplasia without evidence of atypia. No serious adverse events were reported. Interestingly, there were no differences in serum oestradiol levels between the treatment and placebo groups (median oestradiol was >50 pg/mL in all groups). However, the numbers studied were small, with 22 patients being allocated and 18 completing the three cycles or 90–120-day trial [47]. An even more recent randomised, double-blind, placebo-controlled trial of efficacy and tolerability has also demonstrated positive results when UA was administered for 3–6 months, showing good control of bleeding, reduction in fibroid size and improvement in quality of life in the treatment group [48]. Ulipristal has recently successfully completed two phase III clinical trials (PEARL I & II) in Europe demonstrating its efficacy and safety for the treatment of symptomatic uterine fibroids in patients eligible for surgery [49,50]. PEARL I compared treatment with oral UA for up to 13 weeks at a dose of 5 mg per day (96 women) or 10 mg per day (98 women) with placebo (48 women) in patients with fibroids, menorrhagia and anaemia. All patients received iron supplementation. The co-primary efficacy endpoints were control of uterine bleeding and reduction of fibroid volume at week 13, after which patients could undergo surgery. At 13 weeks, uterine bleeding was controlled in 91% of the women receiving 5 mg of UA, 92% of those receiving 10 mg of UA and 19% of those receiving placebo ($P < 0.001$ for the comparison of each dose of ulipristal with placebo). Treatment with UA for 13 weeks effectively controlled excessive bleeding due to uterine fibroids and reduced the size of the fibroids [49]. PEARL II was a double-blind noninferiority trial, which randomly assigned 307 patients with symptomatic fibroids and excessive uterine bleeding to receive 3 months of daily therapy with oral UA (at a dose of either 5 or 10 mg) or once monthly intramuscular injections of the GnRH analogue leuprolide acetate (at a dose of 3.75 mg). The primary outcome was the proportion of patients with controlled bleeding at week 13, with a prespecified noninferiority margin of –20%. Uterine bleeding was controlled in 90% of patients receiving 5 mg of UA, in 98% of those receiving 10 mg, whilst the figure for leuprolide acetate was 89%. Both ulipristal doses were noninferior to once monthly leuprolide acetate in controlling uterine bleeding and were significantly less likely to cause hot flushes [50].

Recently the results of long-term or repeated courses of UA have been published. PEARL III and its extension were long-term, open-label, phase III trials of UA, which were double-blinded and placebo-controlled towards the administration of progestin after the end of each ulipristal treatment course [51]. A total of 209 women with symptomatic fibroids including heavy menstrual bleeding were included. Patients received up to four 3-month courses of UA 10 mg daily, immediately followed by 10-day double-blind treatment with norethisterone acetate (NETA) 10 mg daily or placebo. After the first UA course, amenorrhoea occurred in 79% of women, with median onset (from starting of the treatment) of 4 days (interquartile range, 2–6 days). Median fibroid volume change was –45% (interquartile range, –66% to –25%). Amenorrhoea rates were 89, 88 and 90% for the 131, 119 and 107 women who received treatment courses 2, 3 and 4 respectively. Median times to amenorrhoea were 2, 3 and 3 days for treatment courses 2, 3 and 4 respectively. Median fibroid volume changes from baseline were –63, –67 and –72% after treatment courses 2, 3 and 4 respectively. All endometrial biopsies showed benign histology without hyperplasia. NETA did not affect fibroid volume or endometrial histology. The authors concluded that repeated 3-month UA courses effectively control bleeding and shrink fibroids in patients with symptomatic fibroids [51]. Further data are awaited from the PEARL IV study exploring long-term administration of UA at 5 versus 10 mg daily (in 500 women) in Europe.

Presently the licensed treatment of UA consists of one tablet of 5 mg to be taken orally once daily for up to 3 months. Treatment should be started during the first week of a menstrual cycle. If a patient misses a dose, the patient should take UA as soon as possible. If the dose was missed by >12 hours, the patient should not take the missed dose and simply resume the usual dosing schedule.

CONTRAINDICATIONS AND DRUG INTERACTIONS WITH SPRMS

Contraindications to UA therapy include hypersensitivity to the drug, pregnancy, breastfeeding, genital bleeding of unknown aetiology and uterine, cervical, ovarian or breast cancer. Women are advised not to breastfeed and to discard expressed milk for 36 hours after treatment with UA. Mifepristone treatment is contraindicated in cases of confirmed or suspected ectopic pregnancy or undiagnosed adnexal mass, chronic adrenal failure, concurrent long-term corticosteroid therapy, history of allergy to mifepristone, haemorrhagic disorders or concurrent anticoagulant therapy and inherited porphyrias. Because it is important to have access to appropriate medical care if an emergency develops with mifepristone and misoprostol treatment, this treatment protocol is contraindicated if a patient does not have adequate access to medical facilities equipped to provide emergency treatment for incomplete abortion, blood transfusions and emergency resuscitation during the period from the first visit until discharged by the administering physician.

Hormonal contraceptives and progestogens are likely to reduce UA efficacy by competitive action on the PR, and are therefore not recommended. UA is not recommended for patients receiving drugs such as dabigatran etexilate and digoxin. Liver enzyme inducers such as CYP3A4 inducers (e.g. rifampicin, phenytoin, carbamazepine, ritonavir, St John's Wort) may reduce plasma concentrations of UA and may reduce efficacy. However, liver enzyme inhibitors such as CYP3A4 inhibitors (e.g. ketoconazole, itraconazole, clarithromycin) may increase exposure to UA, although the clinical significance of this is uncertain. Use of UA with antacids, proton pump inhibitors and H2 receptor antagonists, or any other drugs that increase gastric pH may reduce absorption of UA and decrease its efficacy. UA binds to PRs and so may reduce the efficacy of progestogen-containing contraceptives.

Renal impairment is not expected to significantly alter the elimination of UA. In the absence of specific studies, UA is not recommended for patients with severe renal impairment unless the patient is closely monitored. Liver toxicity has not been reported as a feature of mifepristone, asoprisnil or UA. On occasion, long-term mifepristone administration in doses ranging from 5 to 200 mg daily has been associated with transient elevation in hepatic enzymes. For two other SPRMs – onapristone and telapristone (high dose) – clinical trials had to be suspended because of their effects on hepatic enzymes [19]. Hepatic impairment is expected to alter the elimination of UA, resulting in increased exposure. This is considered not to be clinically relevant for patients with mildly impaired liver function. UA is not recommended for use in patients with moderate or severe hepatic impairment unless the patient is closely monitored.

A recent study reported the pregnancy rate after UA therapy for fibroids [52]. This was a retrospective analysis of a series of 52 patients prospectively included in the PEARL II and III trials. Amongst the 52 patients, 21 wished to conceive upon treatment completion. Of these, 15 (71%) women conceived 18 pregnancies. Amongst these 18 pregnancies, 12 resulted in the birth of 13 healthy babies and six ended in early miscarriage. No re-growth of fibroids was observed during pregnancy. There were no maternal complications related to myomas during pregnancy. All the babies were healthy. One infant had an ectopic kidney, but this did not seem to be linked to the treatment. Most deliveries were performed by caesarean section, either because of previous surgery for uterine fibroids or in an emergency context for medical or fetal conditions [52].

ADVERSE EFFECTS ASSOCIATED WITH THE USE OF SPRMS

The vast majority of adverse reactions are mild and these include hot flushes, headache, functional ovarian cysts, vertigo, nausea, acne, sweating, muscle pain and tiredness.

Endometrial hyperplasia and thickening

A National Institute of Health-sponsored workshop evaluated endometrial specimens from women receiving mifepristone, asoprisnil and UA [2,8,53,54]. Pathologists were blinded to agent, dose and exposure interval. It was concluded that there was little evidence of mitosis consistent with the antiproliferative effect of SPRMs. No biopsy demonstrated atypical hyperplasia. Asymmetry of stromal and epithelial growth resulted in prominent cystically dilated glands with admixed oestrogen (mitotic) and progestin (secretory) epithelial effects of a type not encountered in contemporary clinical practice. The panel designated these changes as PRM-associated endometrial changes (PAECs) [2,53,54]. Despite the paucity of mitoses, pathologists may associate the cystic glandular dilatation observed with PRMs with simple hyperplasia and should be aware of the potential diagnostic pitfalls of misdiagnosing hyperplasia in women receiving PRMs [2,55,56]. In another study, biopsies were obtained from 58 premenopausal women participating in clinical trials of the SPRM CBD-4124. Biopsies were obtained at 3 and 6 months, and women were receiving daily doses of oral therapy that ranged from 12.5 to 50 mg. Of the 174 samples, 103 contained histological changes not seen in the normal menstrual cycle [43]. Whereas the majority of the histology was atrophic, novel cystic changes were seen with increasing doses. Cystically dilated glands with mixed secretory and mitotic features were noted. These lesions are not considered to be premalignant and no malignancies were found. It has been suggested that the endometrial thickening in women who use SPRMs is related to cystic glandular dilation and not endometrial hyperplasia [8]. Overall, only about 10% of women on UA in the PEARL studies had endometrial thickness >16 mm. Clinicians detecting endometrial thickening in women treated with PRMs need to be aware that administration of PRMs for >3 months may lead to endometrial thickening. This is related to cystic glandular dilation, not endometrial hyperplasia and pathologists need to be aware of PAECs and avoid misclassifying the appearance as hyperplasia. PAECs are known to always disappear after treatment cessation [49–51].

Although breakthrough bleeding has been reported as one of the side effects of SPRMs, sufficient data assessing their long-term use are not available. It is also argued that these agents are not useful for the treatment of large fibroids as they cause a modest decrease in their size. However, larger clinical trials with varying doses and duration of therapy of PRMs will, in future, be able to provide a definite answer to this question. Given the ubiquitous nature of PR in the human body described earlier in this chapter, long-term studies on the impact of SPRMs are certainly required.

CONCLUSION

SPRMs are a promising group of drugs with applications in several gynaecological conditions such as fibroids, endometriosis, DUB, medical termination of pregnancy and contraception. Their simplicity of administration, minimal side effects and potential low cost render them a preferred modality of treatment in comparison to expensive and invasive therapies. As new research data emerge and large prospective studies are completed, the role of SPRMs will be better defined, especially in relation to their long-term safety and effects on endometrium and reproductive function. The stage is set for definitive clinical trials that should help establish the true role of SPRMs in various gynaecological conditions.

Key points for clinical practice

- SPRMs are PR ligands which possess activity ranging from pure agonist through mixed agonist/antagonist activity to pure antagonist activity.
- Mifepristone, one of the earliest progesterone antagonists, has been commonly used for first trimester medical termination of intrauterine pregnancy with or without misoprostol. It is also used in management of second trimester medical termination of pregnancy and IUFD along with misoprostol.
- A 30 mg ulipristal has been marketed as a single dose emergency contraceptive to be taken within 120 hours of unprotected sexual intercourse. Ulipristal was shown in two large RCTs to be as effective as LNG for emergency contraception when administered within 72 hours of unprotected sexual intercourse.
- UA has been licensed in Europe for use prior to surgery for fibroids.
- Ulipristal has shown efficacy with a significant reduction in uterine bleeding, fibroid volume and improved quality of life, without the side effects associated with other medications such as GnRH agonists in PEARL I and II RCTs.
- Ulipristal treatment consists of one tablet of 5 mg to be taken orally once daily for up to 3 months.
- PEARL III and PEARL III extension studies have also demonstrated the effectiveness of repeated 3-month courses (up to four 3-month courses) of oral ulipristal.
- Endometrial thickening in women treated with SPRMs may be related to cystic glandular dilation, not endometrial hyperplasia, and pathologists need to be aware of PAECs.
- Future trials will define the long-term safety and efficacy of SPRMs in treatment of various gynaecological conditions.

REFERENCES

1. Giangrande PH, McDonnell DP. The A and B isoforms of the human progesterone receptor: two functionally different transcription factors encoded by a single gene. Recent Prog Horm Res 1999; 54:291–313.
2. Spitz IM. Clinical utility of progesterone receptor modulators and their effect on the endometrium. Curr Opin Obstet Gynecol 2009; 21:318–324.
3. Spitz IM. Progesterone receptor antagonists. In: Ottow E, Weinmann H (eds), Nuclear receptors as drug targets. Weinheim: Wiley-VCH, 2008:223-248.
4. Wilkens J, Chwalisz K, Han C, et al. Effects of the selective progesterone receptor modulator asoprisnil on uterine artery blood flow, ovarian activity, and clinical symptoms in patients with uterine leiomyomata scheduled for hysterectomy. J Clin Endocrinol Metab 2008; 93:4664–4671.
5. Spitz IM, Wiehle RD, van As A. Progesterone receptor modulators in endometriosis: a new therapeutic option. In: Garcia-Velasco J, Rizk B (eds). Textbook of endometriosis. New Delhi, India: Jaypee Brothers Medical Publishers Ltd, 2009:225-234.
6. Chabbert-Buffet N, Pintiaux-Kairis A, Bouchard P. Effects of the progesterone receptor modulator VA2914 in a continuous low dose on the hypothalamic–pituitary–ovarian axis and endometrium in normal women: a prospective, randomized, placebo-controlled trial. J Clin Endocrinol Metab 2007; 92:3582–3589.
7. Chwalisz K, Elger W, Stickler T, et al. The effects of one month administration of asoprisnil (J867), a selective progesterone receptor modulator, in normal women. Hum Reprod 2005; 20:1090–1099.
8. Sinai Talaulikar V, Manyonda I. Progesterone and progesterone receptor modulators in the management of symptomatic uterine fibroids. Eur J Obstet Gynecol Reprod Biol 2012; 165:135–140.
9. Maruo T, Matsuo H, Samoto T, et al. Effects of progesterone on uterine leiomyoma growth and apoptosis. Steroids 2000; 65:585–592.
10. Ohara N, Xu Q, Matsuo H, et al. Progesterone and progesterone receptor modulator in uterine leiomyoma growth. In: Maruo T, Mardon H, Stewart C (eds), Translational research in uterine biology. Amsterdam: Elsevier, 2008:161-178.

11. Ohara N, Morikawa A, Chen W, et al. Comparative effects of SPRM asoprisnil (J867) on proliferation, apoptosis, and the expression of growth factors in cultured uterine leiomyoma cells and normal myometrial cells. Reprod Sci 2007; 14(8 Suppl):20–27.

12. Xu Q, Ohara N, Liu J, et al. Progesterone receptor modulator CDB-2914 induces extracellular matrix metalloproteinase inducer in cultured human uterine leiomyoma cells. Mol Hum Reprod 2008; 14:181–191.

13. Morikawa A, Ohara N, Xu Q, et al. Selective progesterone receptor modulator asoprisnil down-regulates collagen synthesis in cultured human uterine leiomyoma cells through up-regulating extracellular matrix metalloproteinase inducer. Hum Reprod 2008; 23:944–951.

14. Yoshida S, Ohara N, Xu Q, et al. Cell-type specific actions of progesterone receptor modulators in the regulation of uterine leiomyoma growth. Semin Reprod Med 2010; 28:260–273.

15. Meng CX, Andersson KL, Bentin-Ley U, et al. Effect of levonorgestrel and mifepristone on endometrial receptivity markers in a three-dimensional human endometrial cell culture model. Fertil Steril 2009; 91:256–264.

16. Wånggren K, Stavreus-Evers A, Olsson C, et al. Regulation of muscular contractions in the human Fallopian tube through prostaglandins and progestogens. Hum Reprod 2008; 23:2359–2368.

17. Ko KKY, Huang VW, Li HWR, et al. An in vitro study of the effect of mifepristone and ulipristal acetate on human sperm functions. Abstract to the 23rd Asian and Oceanic Congress of Obstetrics and Gynaecology. Bangkok: Thailand; 20–23 October 2013.

18. Li HWR, Liao SB, Yeung WSB, et al. Ulipristal acetate may contribute to contraceptive action by its effects on tubal function. Abstract to First Global Conference on Contraception, Reproductive and Sexual Health; 22–25 May 2013.

19. Bouchard P, Chabbert-Buffet N, Fauser BC. Selective progesterone receptor modulators in reproductive medicine: pharmacology, clinical efficacy and safety. Fertil Steril 2011; 96:1175–1189.

20. Kulier R, Kapp N, Gülmezoglu AM, et al. Medical methods for first trimester abortion. Cochrane Database Syst Rev 2011; (11):CD002855.

21. Wildschut H, Both MI, Medema S, et al. Medical methods for mid-trimester termination of pregnancy. Cochrane Database Syst Rev 2011; (1):CD005216.

22. Royal College of Obstetrics and Gynaeocology (RCOG). Late intrauterine fetal death and stillbirth, green-top guideline no. 55. London; RCOG, 2010.

23. Wagaarachchi PT, Ashok PW, Narvekar NN, et al. Medical management of late intrauterine death using a combination of mifepristone and misoprostol. BJOG 2002; 109:443–447.

24. Cabrol D, Dubois C, Cronje H, et al. Induction of labor with mifepristone (RU 486) in intrauterine fetal death. Am J Obstet Gynecol 1990; 163:540–542.

25. British Medical Association and Royal Pharmaceutical Society of Great Britain. British National Formulary (BNF) 58. London: BMJ Publishing Group Ltd and RPS Publishing, 2009.

26. Task Force on Postovulatory Methods of Fertility Regulation. Comparison of three single doses of mifepristone as emergency contraception: a randomized trial. Lancet 1999; 353:697–702.

27. Cheng L, Che Y, Gülmezoglu AM. Interventions for emergency contraception. Cochrane Database Syst Rev 2012; 8:CD001324.

28. Creinin MD, Schlaff W, Archer DF, et al. Progesterone receptor modulator for emergency contraception: a randomized controlled trial. Obstet Gynecol 2006; 108:1089–1097.

29. Glasier AF, Cameron ST, Fine PM, et al. Ulipristal acetate versus levonorgestrel for emergency contraception: a randomised non-inferiority trial and meta-analysis. Lancet 2010; 375:555–562.

30. Stratton P, Hartog B, Hajizadeh N, et al. A single mid-follicular dose of CDB-2914, a new antiprogestin, inhibits folliculogenesis and endometrial differentiation in normally cycling women. Hum Reprod 2000; 15:1092–1099.

31. Brache V, Cochon L, Jesam C, et al. Immediate pre-ovulatory administration of 30 mg ulipristal acetate significantly delays follicular rupture. Hum Reprod 2010; 25:2256–2263.

32. Li HW, Lo SS, Ho PC. Emergency contraception. Best Pract Res Clin Obstet Gynaecol 2014; 28:835–844.

33. Kettel LM, Murphy AA, Morales AJ, et al. Treatment of endometriosis with the antiprogesterone mifepristone (RU486). Fertil Steril 1996; 65:23–28.

34. Chwalisz K, Mattia-Goldberg C, Elger W, et al. Treatment of endometriosis with the novel selective progesterone receptor modulator (SPRM) asoprisnil. Fertil Steril 2004; 82:S83–S84.

35. Chwalisz K, Perez MC, Demanno D, et al. Selective progesterone receptor modulator development and use in the treatment of leiomyomata and endometriosis. Endocr Rev 2005; 26:423–438.

36. Gemzell-Danielsson K, van Heusden AM, Killick SR, et al. Improving cycle control in progestogen-only contraceptive pill users by intermittent treatment with a new anti-progestogen. Hum Reprod 2002; 17:2588–2593.

37. Massai MR, Pavez M, Fuentealba B, et al. Effect of intermittent treatment with mifepristone on bleeding patterns in Norplant implant users. Contraception 2004; 70:47–54.
38. De Leo V, Morgante G, La Marca A, et al. A benefit-risk assessment of medical treatment for uterine leiomyomas. Drug Saf 2002; 25:759–779.
39. Eisinger SH, Meldrum S, Fiscella K, et al. Low-dose mifepristone for uterine leiomyomata. Obstet Gynecol 2003; 101:243–250.
40. Fiscella K, Eisinger SH, Meldrum S. Effect of mifepristone for symptomatic leiomyomata on quality of life and uterine size. Obstet Gynecol 2006; 108:1381–1387.
41. Carbonell Esteve JL, Acosta R, Heredia B, et al. Mifepristone for the treatment of uterine leiomyomas: a randomized controlled trial. Obstet Gynecol 2008; 112:1029–1036.
42. Wiehle RD, Goldberg J, Brodniewicz T, et al. Effects of a new progesterone receptor modulator CDB-4124, on fibroid size and uterine bleeding, US. Obstet Gynecol 2008; 3:17. http://www.touchbriefings.com.
43. Ioffe OB, Zaino RJ, Mutter GL. Endometrial changes from short-term therapy with CDB-4124, a selective progesterone receptor modulator. Mod Pathol 2009; 22:450–459.
44. Brahma PK, Martel KM, Christman GM. Future directions in myoma research. Obstet Gynecol Clin North Am 2006; 33:199–224.
45. Chwalisz K, Lamar Parker R, Williamson S, et al. Treatment of uterine leiomyomas with the novel selective progesterone receptor modulator (SPRM) J867. J Soc Gynecol Investig 2003; 10:636.
46. Chwalisz K, Larsen L, McCrary K, et al. Effects of the novel selective progesterone receptor modulator (SPRM) asoprisnil on bleeding patterns in subjects with leiomyomata. J Soc Gynecol Investig 2004; 11:320A–321A.
47. Levens ED, Potlog-Nahari C, Armstrong AY, et al. CDB-2914 for uterine leiomyomata treatment: a randomized controlled trial. Obstet Gynecol 2008; 111:1129–1136.
48. Nieman LK, Blocker W, Nansel T, et al. Efficacy and tolerability of CDB-2914 treatment for symptomatic uterine fibroids: a randomized, double-blind, placebo-controlled, phase IIb study. Fertil Steril 2011; 95:e1–e2.
49. Donnez J, Tatarchuk TF, Bouchard P, et al. PEARL I Study Group. Ulipristal acetate versus placebo for fibroid treatment before surgery. N Engl J Med 2012; 366:409–420.
50. Donnez J, Tomaszewski J, Vázquez F, et al. PEARL II Study Group. Ulipristal acetate versus leuprolide acetate for uterine fibroids. N Engl J Med 2012; 366:421–432.
51. Donnez J, Vázquez F, Tomaszewski J, et al. PEARL III and PEARL III Extension Study Group. Long-term treatment of uterine fibroids with ulipristal acetate. Fertil Steril 2014; 101:1565-73.e1-18.
52. Luyckx M, Squifflet JL, Jadoul P, et al. First series of 18 pregnancies after ulipristal acetate treatment for uterine fibroids. Fertil Steril 2014; 102:1404-1409.
53. Horne FM, Blithe DL. Progesterone receptor modulators and the endometrium: changes and consequences. Hum Reprod Update 2007; 13:567–580.
54. Mutter GL, Bergeron C, Deligdisch L, et al. The spectrum of endometrial pathology induced by progesterone receptor modulators. Mod Pathol 2008; 21:591–598.
55. Williams AR, Critchley HO, Osei J, et al. The effects of the selective progesterone receptor modulator asoprisnil on the morphology of uterine tissues after 3 months treatment in patients with symptomatic uterine leiomyomata. Hum Reprod 2007; 22:1696–1704.
56. Talaulikar VS, Manyonda IT. Ulipristal acetate: a novel option for the medical management of symptomatic uterine fibroids. Adv Ther 2012; 29:655–663.

Chapter 8

Minimising complications associated with caesarean section

Malcolm Griffiths

INTRODUCTION

Caesarean section (CS) is one of the most commonly performed surgical procedures. In many institutions, over a third of births are by CS. Many women who have previously delivered by CS will make an informed decision for elective repeat caesarean section (ERCS). CS carries significant risks of complications to the woman and her child(ren) both immediately and in the future. Most CS are performed through a lower segment transverse incision (LSCS), and this chapter will review complications associated with this widely adopted technique. It should be remembered, however, that the uterine cavity can also be accessed through a vertical incision made on the uterus either through the upper segment (classical incision) or across both the upper and lower segments (De Lee incision). These latter approaches carry additional risks and are usually restricted to specific indications such as extreme prematurity, abnormal presentations and placentation problems. An in-depth discussion of potential anaesthetic risks falls outside the scope of this chapter, but it is clear that regional anaesthesia is preferred for CS and that antacid prophylaxis should be used in case of a need for general anaesthesia along with other physical precautions against the increased risk of aspiration of gastric contents in pregnancy [1].

Steps to avoid unnecessary CS are likely to reduce the total burden of CS deliveries and associated complications. Measures to avoid unnecessary CS are best founded on evidence-based guidelines [2-4] and quality standards [5], e.g. from National Institute for Health and Care Excellence (NICE) and relate to optimal management in labour, appropriate use of augmentation, correct interpretation of fetal heart rate monitoring, senior obstetrician involvement in decision-making and use of confirmatory tests where fetal compromise is suspected.

This chapter, however, will focus on the intraoperative risks and postoperative complications associated with CS affecting both mother and the baby. Complications that may arise from CS can be categorised into (1) general surgical risks including anaesthetic complications, infection, haemorrhage and thromboembolism and (2) specific surgical risks relating to fetal injury at the time of delivery, damage to adjacent organs/structures

Malcolm Griffiths MD MA FRCOG FFSRH, Department of Obstetrics and Gynaecology, Luton and Dunstable University Hospital, Luton, UK. Email: malcolmgriffiths@nhs.net (for correspondence)

Table 8.1 Serious risks associated with caesarean section (CS)		
	Risk	**Frequency (%)**
Maternal risks	Emergency hysterectomy	0.7–0.8
	No need for further surgery	0.50
	Bladder injury	0.10
	Ureteric injury	0.03
	Death	0.01
Fetal injury	Laceration	2
Future pregnancies	Risk of uterine rupture	0.40
	Antepartum stillbirth	0.40
	Morbidity adherent placenta	0.4–0.8

More detail of the various adverse outcomes, differences between different types of CS and estimated relative rates compared with vaginal birth are available in Tables 4.5 and 4.6 in the current NICE guideline on sections [3,6].

and postpartum haemorrhage (PPH). In addition to these more immediate complications, there may be problems arising from CS in the longer term. These may include problems with healing of the uterine scar and subsequent adverse impacts on reproduction such as risk of stillbirth, reduced fertility and fecundity, increased chance of a morbidly adherent placenta and in turn possible psychological consequences (**Table 8.1**). In addition to maternal complications of CS, there may be adverse consequences for the child. It is now well accepted that short- and medium-term respiratory morbidity is increased in the infant, especially after early elective CS, but less recognised and more contentious are the possible long-term adverse impacts on the child of birth by CS.

GENERAL CONSIDERATIONS

Surgical techniques

There are a range of options concerning surgical techniques for CS and these include choice of skin and abdominal incision, method of uterine entry, mode of fetal delivery (manual/instrumental), use of oxytocic drugs, approach to delivery of the placenta and techniques for uterine, abdominal and skin closure. Hema and Johanson wrote an excellent review [7] of this subject, a number of these issues have also been covered by NICE [3,8] and some elements of the available options were covered in the CAESAR [9] and CORONIS [10] studies. CAESAR specifically addressed the following: single versus double-layer closure of the uterus, closure versus nonclosure of the pelvic peritoneum, restricted versus liberal use of subsheath drain, the main outcome measure being maternal infectious morbidity. The CORONIS [11] study covered a wider range of elements of surgical technique (blunt versus sharp abdominal entry, exteriorisation of the uterus for repair versus intra-abdominal repair, single versus double-layer closure of the uterus, closure versus nonclosure of the peritoneum and different suture materials). No differences were found in either study between any of these comparisons in terms of short-term outcome. Double-layer uterine closure, peritoneal closure or drain use conferred no benefit; omission of these elements did not increase the incidence of early maternal complications, but saved time and resources. Follow-up data from both studies are eagerly awaited to assess longer term outcomes, such as subsequent subfertility, mode of delivery and integrity of the uterine scar in further pregnancies. For example, without knowing the long-term outcomes of single-layer closure, a change in long-established practice may be premature.

Whilst acknowledging the potential risks of CS and taking steps to minimise complications, clinicians and their patients need to be aware that a planned vaginal birth, whether primary or following previous CS, is never without risks; the outcome may be a complicated vaginal birth or an in-labour emergency CS. Consideration of the relative risks of vaginal birth and CS is especially germane when counselling women requesting CS or in those considering vaginal birth after CS (VBAC).

Women with previous caesarean section

Amongst those women who opt to attempt VBAC (sometimes referred to as trial of labour after caesarean), around a quarter will be delivered by intrapartum CS. Both ERCS and intrapartum CS after failed VBAC carry additional risks of complications, when compared to the risks of primary CS. Indeed, the relative risks of complications between ERCS and VBAC attempts are broadly similar [2,3].

Second stage caesarean section

An increasing proportion of CS is done at full dilatation. This subject has recently been reviewed by Vousden et al [12]. Various reasons are suggested for the increasing rate, the main issues being avoidance of more complicated instrumental deliveries and an increased tendency to abandon a trial of instrumental delivery. Whether this is a good or a bad thing is unclear. Certainly some maternal or neonatal complications of difficult instrumental delivery may be avoided, but the downside is the greater risk of maternal or neonatal complications associated with second stage CS. Vousden advises that these risks are not generally increased after an attempted operative vaginal delivery, but that individual patient decisions need to be made by senior obstetricians.

An extension of a LSCS incision, especially at full cervical dilatation, may be difficult to avoid other than by careful, gentle delivery of the presenting part. An issue with second stage CS relates to disimpaction of the fetal head. It is generally accepted that pushing the head up vaginally before CS, particularly after a failed trial of vaginal delivery, may aid delivery of the fetal presenting part at CS. However, difficulties may arise when the head cannot be displaced from the pelvis. The options available to the accoucheur are to employ the 'push' or 'pull' techniques:

- 'Push' requires an additional operator to insert fingers into the vagina and push the head up. It is unwise to delegate this task to an inexperienced assistant unless with detailed directions. The assistant needs to displace the head upwards, ideally providing flexion, using as many fingers as possibly to thereby spread the pressure. Skull fractures have occurred with single finger pressure.
- 'Pull' involves a difficult internal podalic version whereby the feet and breech are delivered first, followed by the trunk and lastly the after-coming head. Risks are of fetal trauma or extension of the incision.

Other techniques including Patwardhan's technique (delivering the shoulders, then trunk breech and lastly the head) are occasionally mentioned, but none have been subject to any appropriate assessment, though at least one group in India has reported positive experience with the technique [13].

The 'Fetal Pillow' has been promoted as an atraumatic device to displace the fetal head upwards. It is inserted by the vagina and only inflated once the mother has been positioned for CS. Papanikolaou et al [14] have reported a small uncontrolled series, from which they concluded that the device was safe and helped in the delivery of the impacted fetal head. Seal and colleagues (in India) have reported a controlled trial. Their report is available only as an abstract on the manufacturer's website but is referred to by Attilakos [15]. This was a randomised study of 202 cases and in the pillow-treated group, operating time, incision to delivery, extension of incision and blood loss were all apparently significantly improved. Vousden [12] also refers to the 'C-snorkel' device which is intended to release a supposed vacuum that prevents disimpaction. Again there is no evidence of efficacy or safety.

Large randomised trials are needed to further evaluate such technologies before they can be recommended for use in routine clinical practice.

Maternal request for caesarean section

Some women request delivery by CS and often the basis for this desire is tocophobia or a previous traumatic vaginal birth [2,3,16]. There is no clear consensus on permitting CS by maternal choice. NICE have recommended that 'For women requesting a CS, if after discussion and offer of support (including perinatal mental health support for women with anxiety about childbirth), a vaginal birth is still not an acceptable option, offer a planned CS' [3]. In the United States, a National Institutes of Health Consensus Conference [17] [reiterated by the American Congress of Obstetricians & Gynecologists (ACOG) [18]] made a series of recommendations:

- In the absence of maternal or fetal indications for caesarean delivery, a plan for vaginal delivery is safe and appropriate and should be recommended.
- The following is recommended in cases in which caesarean delivery on maternal request is planned:
  - Caesarean delivery on maternal request should not be performed before a gestational age of 39 weeks
  - Caesarean delivery on maternal request should not be motivated by the unavailability of effective pain management
  - Caesarean delivery on maternal request particularly is not recommended for women desiring several children, given that the risks of placenta praevia, placenta accreta and gravid hysterectomy increase with each caesarean delivery

Human factors

Consideration of 'human factors' [19] in high risk areas of medicine are thought to minimise the risk of errors by increasing situational awareness [20]. The tools used are checklists, handovers of 'situation, background, assessment, recommendation' [21] with team briefing and debriefing. These can be enhanced by empowering all team members to speak out [22]. Lessons can be learned from practices in other professions such as aviation. An example of a failure of team-working in an acute setting can be viewed at http://www.institute.nhs.uk/safer_care/general/human_factors.html.

Poor workplace behaviours, in particular undermining and bullying of colleagues and team members may negatively impact on team performance and information sharing. Accordingly poor behaviour towards colleagues is necessarily a patient safety issue.

Practitioners, educators, employers and regulatory bodies need to take action to address poor behaviour to avoid harm to patients [23].

Health care professionals should inform and empower their patients, such that they can make autonomous choices as opposed to the traditional paternalistic approach to decision-making. 'Informed choice' is now considered a vital component in maternity care [3], but autonomy is often challenged [24] and in obstetrics is often complicated by issues concerning maternal, paternal and fetal rights. This conflict may lead to complications, resentment and psychological trauma. In obstetrics, we have two patients, mother and baby, both of whom may be at the extremes of physiological reserve, so the potential for error can be great. In addition, several different disciplines may be involved in their care and so the need for good communication and sharing of mental models is of paramount importance to minimise confusion and the risk of harm.

Critical incident reporting and risk management

Derived from the aviation and petrochemical industries, incident reporting and risk management techniques are well established in many areas of clinical practice, especially in maternity care [25,26]. Typically reporting happens after adverse outcomes, but also from near-misses. The aim of these actions is to minimise future complications through learning from previous incidents [27].

Critical incidents need to be notified by staff. Wherever possible, information should be electronically gathered about specific trigger events by existing information technology systems [28].

Some typical triggers for incident reporting related to caesarean section:

- Massive obstetric haemorrhage
- Bladder/ureteric injury
- Prolonged decision-to-delivery interval
- Conversion from regional to general anaesthesia
- Unplanned call for senior assistance
- Previously undiagnosed low-lying placenta
- Post-operative ileus
- Admission to intensive care/high-dependency unit
- Maternal readmission following CS
- Neonatologist called to elective CS
- Unexpected low Apgar scores/low cord pH/admission to neonatal unit
- Fetal injury at CS

Notified events need to be reviewed by appropriate staff in a timely manner. Governance or risk leads need to be willing and able to challenge colleagues' actions and behaviour in a 'no blame' culture. Where system-based issues are identified, changes to practice facilitated by guidelines or updating of existing guidelines needs to be used to drive practice change. Shah et al [28] have shown that there is considerable variability in maternity-related incidents that trigger local reviews. Mahajan [29] anticipates that appropriate reporting systems will 'enhance the level and quality of reporting, and safety culture'. However, it has been emphasised that reporting systems must be easy, e.g. taking <5 seconds to report, be set in a supportive environment and involve online individual feedback [30].

MATERNAL COMPLICATIONS

Haemorrhage

Haemorrhage during or after CS is generally attributable to uterine atony or trauma. The relevant Royal College of Obstetricians and Gynaecologists (RCOG) Green-top guideline [31] refers to '4 Ts': tone, trauma, tissue (retained products of conception/placenta) and thrombin (coagulation issues). An atonic uterus can occur with any birth, but the risk is particularly increased with prolonged labour (odds ratio [OR] 2.0). Both elective and emergency CS are associated with an increased risk of PPH (OR 2.0 and 4.0 respectively) compared with vaginal delivery. It is recognised that CS in advanced labour (particularly at full dilatation and after a failed trial of instrumental delivery) predisposes not only to atony but to trauma through extension of the uterine incision [32].

The RCOG [31] advises active management of the third stage of labour including administering five international units (iu) of Syntocinon intravenously to aid uterine contraction. The routine administration of a 'high-dose' Syntocinon infusions (40 IU in 500 mL of 0.9% saline) has crept into practice, largely uncritically, as a prophylactic measure in both low- and high-risk cases against PPH at CS. Sheehan et al [33] demonstrated that the use of a 40 iu oxytocin infusion in addition to a 5 iu bolus after caesarean delivery reduced the need for additional uterotonic agents, but it did not affect the overall occurrence of major obstetric haemorrhage unless the CS was performed by junior rather than senior obstetric surgeons.

Other haemostatic measures include physical procedures (brace sutures, haemostatic balloons) and pharmacological agents (carboprost, misoprostol). These interventions should be reserved for treatment of PPH and only considered prophylactically in selective high-risk cases.

Infectious morbidity

Infectious complications encompassing wound infection, intra-abdominal sepsis, endometritis, urinary and respiratory tract sepsis are common following CS, but more common following repeat and emergency CS. In an era when antibiotic prophylaxis was less widespread, Henderson and Love [34] reported rates of infectious morbidity approaching 50%. Routine antibiotic prophylaxis at the time of CS has become the norm [35].

Since the introduction of antibiotic prophylaxis for CS, it has largely been given after cord-clamping, intending to avoid exposing the neonate to antibiotics, but at the same time potentially compromising the effectiveness of the prophylaxis; prophylaxis against all other surgical infection relies on preprocedural administration, thereby achieving high blood levels of antibiotics before the potential introduction into the surgical field of pathogens.

More recently, a number of randomised trials have compared pre-CS administration of antibiotics with later administration and these studies have generally confirmed improved reduction in infectious morbidity with no evidence of harm to the neonate. Pre-CS prophylaxis is now recommended [2,3].

Venous thromboembolism

Even in the absence of an inherent risk of venous thromboembolism (VTE) through a personal or family history of thrombophilia, pregnancy confers an increased risk of VTE. Risk increases around the time of birth and is increased by CS and even more so by emergency CS. VTE remains a significant cause of maternal death in the confidential enquiries into maternal deaths [36], although the incidence of VTE has fallen over recent triennia, presumably due to the impact of increased prophylaxis.

RCOG guidance [37] is focussed on risk assessment and risk scoring. Broadly speaking, women undergoing CS considered to be at low risk (i.e. low parity women having an elective CS) are recommended for early mobilisation and antiembolism hosiery. In contrast, higher risk women (i.e. high parity, emergency CS and other risk factors) are recommended to have low molecular weight heparin (LMWH). Very high-risk cases may warrant prophylaxis for longer periods (e.g. up to 6 weeks postnatally). Current guidelines largely fail to consider absolute or even relative risks and none addresses the number of women needed to treat to prevent a VTE event.

Injury to other organs

Organs most often at risk of surgical injury during CS excluding uterine trauma are the adjacent structures: bladder, ureter and bowel [3,6]. These are at greater risk of injury in emergency cases and cases of repeat surgery. Where possible, it is important to anticipate potential difficulty (e.g. previously documented difficult CS, women with other previous complex intra-abdominal surgery, obesity etc.) and arrange for the appropriate personnel to be present such as a senior obstetric surgeon and surgeons from other relevant disciplines, to assist or perform the surgery. Indeed, in exceptional circumstances, the risk of out-of-hours emergency CS might be considered so high as to justify earlier elective delivery by CS to minimise the likelihood of spontaneous labour.

Bowel

Bowel preparation is not usually needed, but consultation with a colorectal surgeon is advisable in women with a history of extensive prior bowel surgery. Particular issues arise with delivery of women with an ileal pouch following colectomy for inflammatory bowel disease, and in such cases antenatal review and immediate postoperative review by a coloproctologist should be arranged.

Urinary tract

Bladder injuries are a particular risk with second stage and repeat CS, especially if the bladder is adherent to the lower uterine segment. Routine practice is to insert an indwelling urethral catheter immediately prior to surgery. Where there is a suspicion of bladder injury, instillation via the catheter of methylene blue may allow reassurance or aid identification of a defect.

Ureter is at the greatest risk of injury with scar rupture or if the CS incision extends laterally and/or downwards. Though the ureter is only very rarely involved in such injuries, it may be included in a misplaced suture. Closing the extension is occasionally problematic as it can be difficult to achieve haemostasis. The general advice is to identify the ureter, so it can be deviated away from the operative field to minimise inadvertent injury. Ideal though these manoeuvres may be, it is not always easy due to distorted anatomy, oedematous tissues and massive bleeding. A senior obstetrician needs to be involved in such cases. Where doubt remains over ureteric integrity, advice may be sought from an urologist or postoperative contrast imaging of the lower ureter be arranged. Often where a ureter is snagged by a suture, it may be possible to maintain integrity by antegrade or retrograde ureteric stenting early in the puerperium.

Adhesion prevention

Any intra-abdominal surgery may result in adhesion formation. Such adhesions may complicate future pelvic surgery and in particular repeat CS [38,39]. Adhesions post-CS may become apparent at the time of subsequent pelvic surgery or manifest themselves through subsequent presenting symptoms such as dyspareunia, chronic pelvic pain, small bowel obstruction and infertility [16,40].

Avoidance of adhesions has traditionally been based on 'good surgical technique' involving minimising tissue trauma, ensuring haemostasis, avoiding infection and using suture material that limits foreign-body reaction. Beyond this, efforts have involved hydroflotation (with or without heparinoids), use of nonsteroidal anti-inflammatory drugs (NSAIDs) or the use of specific adhesion barriers. Evidence concerning hydroflotation and NSAIDs are at best conflicting. The literature concerning adhesion barriers appears superficially more positive. Certainly, the various manufacturers strongly promote their use. However, such recommendations are often based on extrapolation from the use of such barriers in other surgical settings and not CS. The only adhesion barrier that has been studied for CS patients is Seprafilm; one often quoted small study [41] is written in Japanese and not readily accessible, but others supported by the manufacturers of the carboxymethylcellulose adhesion barrier, Seprafilm [42] gave details of the Japanese study in a narrative review. No postoperative adhesions were observed in the six women who had Seprafilm where follow-up was available compared to 12/22 controls. However, no information was given as to blinding of observers or details of how adhesions were assessed. A further study using Seprafilm has been carried out [43]; and showed no benefit, i.e. prior use of this adhesion barrier was not associated with decreased time to delivery, total operative time or complications during repeat CS.

A Cochrane review concerning the use of 'barrier agents' in gynaecological surgery [45] concluded that the absorbable adhesion barrier Interceed reduced the incidence of adhesion formation following laparoscopy and laparotomy, but insufficient data are available to support its routine use to improve subsequent pregnancy rates. Gore-Tex may be superior to Interceed in preventing adhesion formation, but its usefulness is limited by the need for suturing and later removal. No evidence was identified supporting the effectiveness of Seprafilm and fibrin sheet placement in preventing adhesion formation.

Psychological sequelae

There is a general presumption that in-labour and unexpected CS may impact negatively on maternal satisfaction and subsequent psychological sequelae. However, a systematic review [46] did not establish a link between CS and postpartum depression. A randomised trial of VBAC versus ERCS [47] found no difference between the two groups in terms of psychological outcome.

'Debriefing' after adverse outcome or unplanned interventions is generally encouraged [48] and promoted widely in RCOG Green-top guidelines [for example, 31]. However, a structured literature review [49] concerning 'postnatal debriefing interventions' concluded that 'whilst women valued opportunities to discuss their birth, evidence to support the content and timing of service provision and effectiveness of this was lacking', further that 'it might be appropriate to consider offering women an opportunity to discuss their childbirth experience and to differentiate this discussion from the offer of a formal debriefing, which is unsupported by evidence.'

An RCOG Query Bank response [50] concludes that 'psychological debriefing' should not be implemented into practice. This view is supported by a systematic review [49] that showed no benefit of debriefing after childbirth in terms of transient psychological problems of depression, anxiety, psychosis and post-traumatic stress disorder (PTSD). Debriefing generally has not been shown to reduce incidence or severity of PTSD [51].

Future stillbirth

An increased risk of antepartum stillbirth has been shown in population based data from Scotland following prior birth by CS [52-55], but these findings have been contradicted by a similar study from Canada. Other negative studies have been published from Bavaria [56] and the United States [57]; however, one group in Missouri [58] found no increased risk in white women, but that there might be an increased risk in black women. Apart from avoiding unnecessary CS, there appears to be no appropriate intervention to address any purported risk; the incidence is too low to consider any form of increased fetal surveillance.

FETAL COMPLICATIONS

Timing of caesarean section and prophylactic corticosteroids

Timing of delivery by CS will often be determined by the maternal condition or by concerns over the fetal condition. However, the impact of even relative prematurity is now well established [59]. With elective CS, there is necessarily a compromise between minimising the risks of relative prematurity and the impact on neonatal respiratory function against the likelihood of spontaneous onset of labour. The onset of labour prior to a planned CS may give rise to concerns over the risk of scar rupture or more frequently the need to perform an in-labour CS, with greater inherent risks especially if labour is well established or delivery needs to be out-of-hours. Morrison et al [59] found the incidence of respiratory distress syndrome (RDS) fell from 42.3 per 1000 at 38 weeks to 17.8 per 1000 at 39 weeks.

The NICE (based on the RCOG Sentinel CS study [60]) concluded that only 18% of women booked for an elective CS after 39 weeks would labour before 39 weeks and on this basis advises that [8]: 'The risk of respiratory morbidity is increased in babies born by CS before labour, but this risk decreases significantly after 39 weeks. Therefore, planned CS should not routinely be carried out before 39 weeks.'

The RCOG [61] has also recommended the use of prophylactic corticosteroids to minimise the risk of RDS in the neonatal period for women having elective CS before 39 weeks. This advice though is based solely on a single study [62]. The methodology and conclusions of this study, especially the end points used (admission to neonatal intensive care unit and no occurrence of RDS), have been criticised, in particular in an accompanying editorial [63] and by the authors of another study which showed no benefit from steroids on the incidence of RDS after 34 weeks [64]. A Cochrane Review [65] concluded that more studies with larger samples are needed to investigate the effect of prophylactic steroids prior to elective CS at term on the incidence of neonatal complications per se. Also more data and longer follow-up would be needed for potential harms and complications. Whenever possible it would seem wise to delay elective CS until 39 weeks. Whenever possible it would seem wise to delay elective CS until 39 weeks. However, many women with diabetes or gestational diabetes often require elective CS before 39 weeks [66]. Thus, the routine administration of prophylactic corticosteroids has major clinical and resource implications in this group of women and is contentious in the absence of compelling evidence for neonatal benefit.

Scalpel laceration

The NICE [3] currently acknowledges a risk of scalpel laceration and recommends that 'Women who are having a CS should be informed that the risk of fetal lacerations is about 2%'. This estimate is largely based on a small survey in a single UK hospital [67], although others have reported such injuries with varying estimates [68,69]. The NICE statement also seems to imply acceptance of such injuries, but it is arguable that such lacerations are entirely avoidable using appropriate techniques. Hema and Johanson [7] state that fetal injury at CS is not uncommon and is often unreported and that scalp wounds should not be considered as 'expected' complications. The long-term sequelae of such lacerations have been reported [70].

Operative technique at the time of CS is important to minimise the risk of fetal injury. Lanneau et al [71] describe opening the lower segment as a sharp incision using the scalpel in the midline performed down to the level of the fetal membranes, with care being made not to incise the membranes. Story and Patterson-Brown [72] advise to leave the membranes intact to avoid the risk of cutting the baby and to maintain the liquor until the uterine incision is completed with particular attention to avoid cutting the baby where the membranes have already ruptured, in cases of oligohydramnios, breech presentations, advanced labour or after repeat CS. In the UK, the NHS Litigation Authority [73] stated that fetal scalpel injuries would be regarded as substandard care unless there were particular extenuating circumstances.

The 'blunt' scalpel reported in Japan [74] no longer seems to be available. Other techniques to avoid fetal lacerations have been described [75], including use of blunt instrumentation and moving the uterine wall away from the fetus prior to incision. Gerber [76] as long ago as 1974 advocated elevating the lower segment before opening with a clamp or forceps. Others use a hybrid of initial sharp uterine incision using a scalpel to score the myometrium followed by more controlled entry using either dissecting scissors or blunt approaches with instruments or digitally.

Hazards to the child of prelabour caesarean section

Sinha and Bewley have raised concerns about the physiological impact on the child who is born without having been exposed to labour [77,78]. They highlight new evidence of immunological and metabolic differences induced by obstetric interventions and conclude that 'normal babies would indeed "choose" labour'. They highlight concerns over routine early cord-clamping, lower breastfeeding rates, mother–baby bonding and an increased rate of type-2 diabetes associated with 'PLCS' (prelabour CS) [77].

Another group has demonstrated an increased risk of childhood obesity associated with delivery by CS after having adjusted for birth weight, gender, parental body mass, family sociodemographics, gestational factors and infant feeding patterns [79]. A series of meta-analyses have shown associations between birth by CS and childhood-onset type 1 diabetes [80], asthma [81] and obesity [82].

Sinha and Bewley do acknowledge the need for further research whilst advising that mothers be 'informed of all the evidence' before consenting to CS, and that 'obstetricians should consider the physiological benefit of labour (even if it results in CS) to optimise neonatal outcome when making individual decisions with women' [78]. Indeed, Hyde and Modi [83] have argued for a randomised controlled trial to address the long-term effects of birth by CS.

Key points for clinical practice

- Avoid unnecessary CS by following evidence-based guidelines and ensuring optimal management in labour, appropriate use of augmentation, correct interpretation of fetal heart rate monitoring, senior obstetrician involvement in decision-making and use of confirmatory tests where fetal compromise is suspected.
- Single-layer uterine closure and other modifications to surgical technique for CS have been shown not to be associated with adverse short-term outcomes, but follow-up studies are required to determine impact on long-term outcomes—especially the risk of scar rupture in future pregnancies.
- Maternal request for CS should ideally be addressed as early as possible in pregnancy and considered in the context of advice from bodies such as ACOG and NICE.
- Human factors, incident reporting and poor workplace behaviours should routinely be addressed in clinical settings.
- Antibiotic prophylaxis should be recommended for CS and ideally administered preoperatively. Prophylaxis against VTE including possible LMWH should be recommended based on perioperative risk assessment.
- There is no evidence for the use of adhesion-barrier agents outside clinical trials.
- A link between CS and postpartum depression has not been established. No benefit has been shown for debriefing after obstetric interventions in terms of subsequent mental health outcome.
- The link between CS and subsequent stillbirth remains controversial—there appears to be no appropriate intervention to address any purported risk; the incidence is too low to consider any form of increased fetal surveillance.
- Whenever possible, delay elective CS until 39 weeks. The evidence to justify widespread prophylactic corticosteroids close to term is weak and difficult to justify.
- Fetal scalpel injuries would be regarded as substandard care unless there were particular extenuating circumstances.

REFERENCES

1. Dresner MR, Freeman JM. Anaesthesia for caesarean section. Best Pract Res Clin Obstet Gynaecol 15:127–143.
2. Gholitabar M, Ullman R, James D, et al. Caesarean section: summary of updated NICE guidance. BMJ 2011; 343:d7108. doi: 10.1136/bmj.d7108.
3. National Institute for Health and Clinical Excellence (NICE) and National Collaborating Centre for Women's and Children's Health (NCCWC). London; NICE and NCCWC, 2011.
4. National Collaborating Centre for Women's and Children's Health (NCCWC) and National Institute for Health and Clinical Excellence (NICE). Intrapartum care of healthy women and their babies during childbirth. London; NCCWC and NICE, 2007.
5. National Institute for Health and Clinical Excellence (NICE). Quality standard for caesarean section. London; NCIE, 2013.
6. Royal College of Obstetricians and Gynaecologists (RCOG). Obtaining valid consent. Clinical governance advice. London; RCOG, 2014:6.
7. Hema KR, Johanson R. Techniques for performing caesarean section. Best Pract Res Clin Obstet Gynaecol 2001; 15:17–47.

8. National Institute for Health and Clinical Excellence (NICE) and National Collaborating Centre for Women's and Children's Health (NCCWC). Caesarean section. London: NICE, 2004.
9. The CAESAR Study Collaborative Group. Caesarean section surgical techniques: a randomised factorial trial (CAESAR). BJOG 2010; 117:1366–1376.
10. The CORONIS Collaborative Group. Caesarean section surgical techniques (CORONIS): a fractional, factorial, unmasked, randomised controlled trial. Lancet 2013; 382:234–248.
11. The CORONIS Collaborative Group. CORONIS - International study of caesarean section surgical techniques: the follow-up study. BMC Pregnancy Childbirth 2013; 13:215.
12. Vousden N, Cargill Z, Briley A, et al. Caesarean section at full dilatation: incidence, impact and current management. J Obstet Gynaecol 2014; 16:199–205.
13. Saha PK, Gulati R, Goel P, et al. Second stage caesarean section: evaluation of Patwardhan technique. J Clin Diagn Res 2014; 8:93–95.
14. Papanikolaou N, Tillisi A, Louay L, et al. Reducing complications related to caesarean section (CS) in second stage: UK experience in the use of fetal disimpacting system (FDS). Int J Gynecol Obstet 2009; 107:S304.
15. Attilakos G, Draycott T, Gale D, et al. ROBuST: RCOG operative birth simulation training: course manual. Cambridge; Cambridge University Press, 2013.
16. Goodin M, Griffiths M. Caesarean section on demand. Obstet Gynaecol Reprod Med 22:368–370.
17. NIH State of the Science Conference: cesarean delivery on maternal request. Adv Neonatal Care 2006; 6:171–172.
18. American College of Obstetricians and Gynecologists. ACOG committee opinion no. 559: cesarean delivery on maternal request. Obstet Gynecol 2013; 121:904–907.
19. Dalton D, Moran S. Human factors and safety culture in healthcare. London; The Health Foundation, 2013:1-7.
20. Bleetman A, Sanusi S, Dale T, et al. Human factors and error prevention in emergency medicine. Emerg Med J 2012; 29:389–393.
21. Leonard M, Graham S, Bonacum D. The human factor: the critical importance of effective teamwork and communication in providing safe care. BMJ Qual Saf 2004; 13(Suppl 1):i85–i90.
22. Carthey J, Clarke J. Implementing human factors in healthcare. London; Patient Safety First, 2014.
23. Rosenstein AH, O'Daniel M. Disruptive behavior and clinical outcomes: perceptions of nurses and physicians: nurses, physicians, and administrators say that clinicians' disruptive behavior has negative effects on clinical outcomes. Am J Nurs 2005; 105: 54-64.
24. Beckmann C. Ethics in obstetrics and gynecology. In: Beckmann C (ed.), Obstetrics and gynecology Cfms edition. Philadelphia; Lippincott Williams & Wilkins, 2013: 23–28.
25. Vincent C. Incident reporting and patient safety. BMJ 2007; 334:51.
26. Vincent CA, Martin T, Ennis M. Obstetric accidents: the patient's perspective. Br J Obstet Gynaecol 1991; 98:390–395.
27. Woloshynowych M, Rogers S, Taylor-Adams S, et al. The investigation and analysis of critical incidents and adverse events in healthcare. Health Technol Assess 2005; 9:158.
28. Shah A, Mohamed-Ahmed O, McClymont C, et al. Conditions triggering local incident reviews in UK hospital maternity units: a national survey. JRSM Open 2014; 5:2054270414528898.
29. Mahajan RP. Critical incident reporting and learning. Br J Anaesth 2010; 105:69–75.
30. Bolsin SN, Colson M, Patrick A, et al. Critical incident reporting and learning. Br J Anaesth 2010; 105:698.
31. Royal College of Obstetrics and Gynaecology (RCOG). Prevention and management of postpartum haemorrhage, green-top guideline no. 52. London; RCOG, 2009:1-24.
32. Murphy DJ, Liebling RE, Verity L, et al. Early maternal and neonatal morbidity associated with operative delivery in second stage of labour: a cohort study. Lancet 2001; 358:1203–1207.
33. Sheehan SR, Montgomery AA, Carey M, et al. Oxytocin bolus versus oxytocin bolus and infusion for control of blood loss at elective caesarean section: double blind, placebo controlled, randomised trial. BMJ 2011; 343:d4661.
34. Henderson E, Love EJ. Incidence of hospital-acquired infections associated with caesarean section. J Hosp Infect 1995; 29:245–255.
35. Smaill F, Hofmeyr GJ. Antibiotic prophylaxis for cesarean section. Cochrane Database Syst Rev 2002; (3):CD000933.
36. Saving Mothers' Lives: Reviewing maternal deaths to make motherhood safer: 2006–2008. BJOG 2011; 118:1–203.
37. Royal College of Obstetrics and Gynaecology (RCOG). Thrombosis and Embolism during Pregnancy and the Puerperium, Reducing the Risk, green-top guideline no. 37a. London; RCOG, 2009;1-35.

38. Lyell DJ. Adhesions and perioperative complications of repeat cesarean delivery. Am J Obstet Gynecol 205:S11–S18.
39. Clark EAS, Silver RM. Long-term maternal morbidity associated with repeat cesarean delivery. Am J Obstet Gynecol 2011; 205:S2–S10.
40. Gonzalez-Quintero VH, Cruz-Pachano FE. Preventing adhesions in obstetric and gynecologic surgical procedures. Rev Obstet Gynecol 2009; 2:38–45.
41. Fushiki H, Ikoma T, Kobayashi H, et al. [Efficacy of Seprafilm as an adhesion prevention barrier in cesarean sections]. Obstet Gynecol Treat [Japanese] 2005; 91:557–561.
42. Diamond MP, Burns EL, Accomando D, et al. Seprafilm adhesion barrier: (2) a review of the clinical literature on intraabdominal use. Gynecol Surg 2012; 9:247–257.
43. Edwards RK, Ingersoll M, Gerkin RD, et al. Carboxymethylcellulose adhesion barrier placement at primary cesarean delivery and outcomes at repeat cesarean delivery. Obstet Gynecol 2014; 123:923–928.
45. Ahmad G, Duffy JM, Farquhar C, et al. Barrier agents for adhesion prevention after gynaecological surgery. Cochrane Database Syst Rev 2008; (2):CD000475.
46. Carter FA, Frampton CMA, Mulder RT. Cesarean section and postpartum depression: a review of the evidence examining the link. Psychosom Med 2006; 68:321–330.
47. Law LW, Pang MW, Chung TK-H, et al. Randomised trial of assigned mode of delivery after a previous cesarean section––impact on maternal psychological dynamics. J Matern Fetal Neonatal Med 2010; 23:1106–1113.
48. Tan M, Mustafa H. PA.33 How well are we debriefing patients after interventional deliveries? A patient safety improvement project. Arch Dis Child Fetal Neonatal Ed 2014; 99 (Suppl 1).
49. Rowan C, Bick D, Bastos MHdS. Postnatal debriefing interventions to prevent maternal mental health problems after birth: exploring the gap between the evidence and UK policy and practice. Worldviews Evid Based Nurs 2007; 4:97–105.
50. Royal College of Obstetricians and Gynaecologists (RCOG). Debriefing after adverse obstetric outcome–– query bank. London; RCOG, 2011:1-9.
51. Rose SC, Bisson J, Churchill R, et al. Psychological debriefing for preventing post traumatic stress disorder (PTSD). Cochrane Database Syst Rev 2002; (2):CD000560.
52. Smith GCS, Pell JP, Cameron AD, et al. Risk of perinatal death associated with labor after previous cesarean delivery in uncomplicated term pregnancies. JAMA 2002; 287:2684–2690.
53. Smith GC, Pell JP, Dobbie R. Caesarean section and risk of unexplained stillbirth in subsequent pregnancy. Lancet 2003; 362:1779–1784.
54. Smith GC, Wood A. Previous caesarean and the risk of antepartum stillbirth. BJOG 2008; 115:1458.
55. Smith GC. Predicting antepartum stillbirth. Curr Opin Obstet Gynecol 2006; 18:625–630.
56. Franz MB, Lack N, Schiessl B, et al. Stillbirth following previous cesarean section in Bavaria/Germany 1987-2005. Arch Gynecol Obstet 2009; 279:29–36.
57. Bahtiyar MO, Julien S, Robinson JN, et al. Prior cesarean delivery is not associated with an increased risk of stillbirth in a subsequent pregnancy: analysis of U.S. perinatal mortality data, 1995-1997. Am J Obstet Gynecol 2006; 195:1373v1378.
58. Salihu HM, Sharma PP, Kristensen S, et al. Risk of stillbirth following a cesarean delivery: black-white disparity. Obstet Gynecol 2006; 107:383–390.
59. Morrison JJ, Rennie JM, Milton PJ. Neonatal respiratory morbidity and mode of delivery at term: influence of timing of elective caesarean section. Br J Obstet Gynaecol 1995; 102:101–106.
60. Thomas J, Callwood A, Brocklehurst P, et al. The National Sentinel Caesarean Section Audit. BJOG 2000; 107:579–580.
61. RCOG. Antenatal corticosteroids to reduce neonatal morbidity, green-top guideline no. 7. London: RCOG; 2010. 1-13.
62. Stutchfield P, Whitaker R, Russell I, on behalf of the Antenatal Steroids for Term Elective Caesarean Section (ASTECS) Research Team. Antenatal betamethasone and incidence of neonatal respiratory distress after elective caesarean section: pragmatic randomised trial. BMJ 2005; 331:662.
63. Steer PJ. Giving steroids before elective caesarean section. Br Med J 2005; 331:645–646.
64. Ana Maria FP, Isabela CC, Jailson BC, et al. Effectiveness of antenatal corticosteroids in reducing respiratory disorders in late preterm infants: randomised clinical trial. BMJ 2011; 342:d1696.
65. Sotiriadis A, Makrydimas G, Papatheodorou S, et al. Corticosteroids for preventing neonatal respiratory morbidity after elective caesarean section at term. Cochrane Database Syst Rev 2009; (4):CD006614.
66. National Institute for Health and Clinical Excellence (NICE). Diabetes in pregnancy: management of diabetes and its complications from pre-conception to the postnatal period. London: NICE 2008.

67. Wiener JJ, Westwood J. Fetal lacerations at caesarean section. J Obstet Gynaecol 2002; 22:23–24.

68. Okaro JM, Anya SE. Accidental incision of the fetus at caesarian section. Niger J Med 2004; 13:56v58.

69. Aburezq H, Chakrabarty KH, Zuker RM. Iatrogenic fetal injury. Obstet Gynecol 2005; 106:1172–1174.

70. Gajjar K, Spencer C. Fetal laceration injury during cesarean section and its long-term sequelae: a case report. Am J Obstet Gynecol 2009; 201:e5–e7.

71. Lanneau GS, Muffley P, Magann EF. Cesarean birth: surgical techniques. In: Sciarra JJ (ed.), Gynecology and obstetrics. Philadelphia; J.B. Lippincott, 2004.

72. Story L, Patterson-Brown S. Cesarean deliveries: indications, techniques and complications. Best practice in labour and delivery. Cambridge; Cambridge University Press, 2009.

73. NHS Litigation Authority (NHSLA). Risk Management in Practice Review, Issue 34. London; Willis Ltd, 2006.

74. Ishii S, Endo M. Blunt-edged, notched scalpel for Cesarean incision. Obstet Gynecol 1999; 94:469–470.

75. Fetal Lacerations Associated with Cesarean Section. 2004. PA PSRS Patient Saf Advis 2004 Dec;1:9–10.

76. Gerber GH. Accidental incision of the fetus during cesarean section delivery. Int J Gynaecol Obstet 1974; 12:46–48.

77. Sinha A, Bewley S, McIntosh T. Myth: babies would choose prelabour caesarean section. Semin Fetal Neonatal Med 2011; 16:247–253.

78. Sinha A, Bewley S. The harmful consequences of prelabour caesarean section on the baby. Obstet Gynaecol Reprod Med 2012;22:54–56.

79. Blustein J, Attina T, Liu M, et al. Association of caesarean delivery with child adiposity from age 6 weeks to 15 years. Int J Obes 2013; 37:900–906.

80. Cardwell CR, Stene LC, Joner G, et al. Caesarean section is associated with an increased risk of childhood-onset type 1 diabetes mellitus: a meta-analysis of observational studies. Diabetologia 2008; 51:726–735.

81. Thavagnanam S, Fleming J, Bromley A, et al A meta-analysis of the association between Caesarean section and childhood asthma. Clin Exp Allergy 2008; 38:629–633.

82. Li H, Zhou Y, Liu J. The impact of cesarean section on offspring overweight and obesity: a systematic review and meta-analysis. Int J Obes 2013; 37:893–899.

83. Hyde MJ, Modi N. The long-term effects of birth by caesarean section: the case for a randomised controlled trial. Early Hum Dev 2012; 88:943–949.

Chapter 9

Changing practices in the management of first-trimester miscarriage

Maya Al-Memar, Shyamaly D Sur

INTRODUCTION

Miscarriage is the most common pregnancy complication, and it is defined as the loss of a pregnancy before 24 completed weeks' gestation. First-trimester miscarriage refers to pregnancy loss before 12+6 weeks' gestation, whilst mid-trimester miscarriage denotes to loss of a pregnancy between 13 and 24 weeks' gestation. In this chapter, we will focus on the former. Miscarriage rarely results in significant physical morbidity; however, it can be associated with serious social and psychological implications to the mother [1]. It is, therefore, crucial that diagnosis of miscarriage is accurate and timely and that women suffering miscarriage are treated compassionately and with sensitivity. The diagnosis, terminology and treatment of miscarriage should be evidence-based and where possible standardised to aid effective management of this common condition.

Incidence

Miscarriage is estimated to occur in 10-20% of clinical pregnancies, although this may be an underestimate because women may miscarry spontaneously before a clinical diagnosis is made. It is thought that first-trimester miscarriage accounts for approximately 50,000 inpatient admissions to hospitals in the UK annually [2].

Terminology

Classification of miscarriage is clinically important because the type and stage of first-trimester loss influences the relative success rates and treatment outcomes of the available management options. Miscarriage can be classified into three groups.

Maya Al-Memar BSc MRCOG, Early Pregnancy and Acute Gynaecology Unit, Queen Charlotte's and Chelsea Hospital, London, UK

Shyamaly D Sur PhD MA MRCOG, Early Pregnancy and Acute Gynaecology Unit, Queen Charlotte's and Chelsea Hospital, London, UK. Email: Shyamaly.Sur@imperial.nhs.uk (for correspondence)

Complete miscarriage

Pregnant women who have bled heavily, and have had an ultrasound scan which shows an empty uterus with no retained products of conception (RPOC), may be diagnosed with a complete miscarriage provided that an intrauterine gestation sac (GS) has previously been identified on ultrasound imaging. Where a pelvic ultrasound scan has not previously been performed or if the findings were inconclusive, the pregnancy must be considered to be of unknown location, irrespective of the history, and further assessment with serial biochemical tests should be undertaken. It has been reported that in 5.9% of cases with a history suggesting passage of products of conception, an ectopic pregnancy has been subsequently diagnosed [3,4].

Once the diagnosis of a complete miscarriage has been made, no further management is required unless the patient continues to have clinical symptoms or if the miscarriage occurs in a series of recurrent pregnancy losses.

Missed miscarriage

A diagnosis of a missed miscarriage can be made where a transvaginal ultrasound scan (TVS) shows a miscarriage, according to the diagnostic criteria shown in **Table 9.1**, and the GS remains within the uterine cavity (**Figures 9.1** and **9.2**). A missed miscarriage may be associated with vaginal bleeding such that the diagnosis is made following an unscheduled early pelvic ultrasound scan. However, a significant proportion of missed miscarriages are diagnosed at the time of a routine dating scan in asymptomatic women [5].

Table 9.1 Diagnosis of miscarriage based on ultrasound findings both at initial scan and those that require interval ultrasound scan for diagnosis [18]		
Ultrasound findings	**Diagnosis**	**Repeat interval**
An empty endometrial cavity with no evidence of retained products of conception (hyperechoic irregular tissues within the uterine cavity) in a woman who had previously undergone a transvaginal ultrasound scan which showed a viable intrauterine pregnancy, pregnancy of uncertain viability, delayed miscarriage, empty sac or incomplete miscarriage	Complete miscarriage	
The presence of heterogeneous, hyperechoic irregular tissues within the uterine cavity	Incomplete miscarriage	
CRL >7 mm with no visible fetal heart activity (**Figure 9.1**)	Missed miscarriage	N/A
MSD ≥25 mm with no visible yolk sac or fetal pole (**Figure 9.2**)	Missed miscarriage	(For measurements near the decision boundaries, a second operator should check findings)
CRL <7 mm and no visible heartbeat (**Figure 9.3**)	PUV	Minimum 7 days If no heartbeat visualised, miscarriage
Empty gestational sac (GS) with MSD <25 mm (**Figure 9.4**)	PUV	Minimum 14 days If no embryo seen, miscarriage
GS with yolk sac but no fetal pole (**Figure 9.5**)	PUV	Minimum 11 days
CRL, crown rump length; MSD, mean sac diameter; PUV, pregnancy of uncertain viability.		

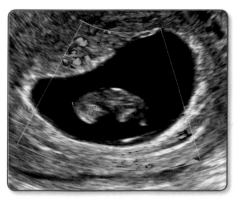

Figure 9.1 Missed miscarriage. The crown rump length is >7 mm and no fetal heartbeat was visualised on transvaginal ultrasound scan.

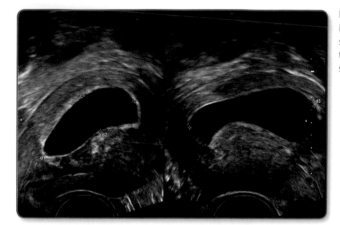

Figure 9.2 Missed miscarriage. There is an empty gestation sac, the mean sac diameter (measured as the mean of three orthogonal measurements of the sac) of which is >25 mm.

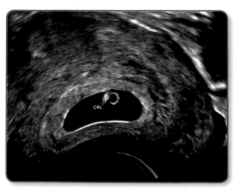

Figure 9.3 Pregnancy of unknown viability with fetal pole. The crown rump length of this fetal pole is 2 mm and there is no fetal heartbeat. A diagnosis of miscarriage cannot be made on the basis of this ultrasound scan and a repeat transvaginal ultrasound scan should be arranged after 7 days.

Incomplete miscarriage

This was previously diagnosed on the basis of an open internal cervical os, but with the widespread adoption of TVS, this type of miscarriage is diagnosed where heterogeneous irregular tissue is seen within the uterine cavity on TVS compatible with RPOC. Measurements of endometrial thickness are not helpful and diagnosis is now based on the subjective impression of the examiner [6]. The application of colour Doppler to assess

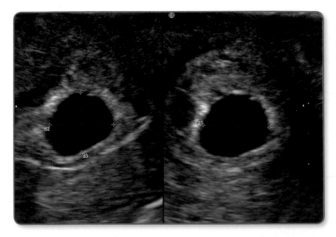

Figure 9.4 Pregnancy of unknown viability. The empty gestation sac has a mean sac diameter of <25 mm, and therefore a diagnosis of miscarriage cannot be made and the patient should be offered a repeat transvaginal ultrasound scan in 14 days.

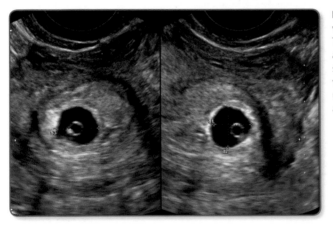

Figure 9.5 Pregnancy of unknown viability with gestation sac and yolk sac. This transvaginal ultrasound scan shows an intrauterine gestation sac with a yolk sac. This is a pregnancy of unknown viability and a repeat transvaginal ultrasound scan should be arranged after a minimum of 11 days.

vascularity of the tissue can be used to help guide management as significant vascularity is more suggestive of retained tissue, as opposed to blood clot [6].

Aetiology

The majority of first-trimester miscarriages are secondary to chromosomal abnormality [7]. Maternal factors that may be associated with recurrent pregnancy loss include maternal age, maternal medical conditions (including antiphospholipid syndrome, polycystic ovarian syndrome and diabetes), congenital uterine abnormalities and smoking [8-13].

DIAGNOSIS OF MISCARRIAGE

Normal early pregnancy

Pregnancy is identified clinically following spontaneous conception after a missed menstrual period and positive urinary pregnancy test. Gestational dating is calculated from the last menstrual period. A TVS at 4 weeks' gestation demonstrates a thickened endometrium. By 5 weeks' gestation, the intrauterine GS is usually visualised as a small empty fluid collection with rounded edges. It is located within the uterine cavity in the central echogenic portion of the endometrium known as the decidual ring. During the fifth week, the yolk sac appears as a 3–5 mm circular structure, usually being seen within the GS. The embryo can be first seen at 5+5 weeks' gestation near the yolk sac and the embryonic heart pulsation visible shortly thereafter [14].

Miscarriage

The accurate diagnosis of miscarriage is of paramount importance because an erroneous diagnosis can have adverse consequences such as terminating a viable pregnancy or failing to detect an ectopic pregnancy. High-resolution TVS is essential in the diagnosis of miscarriage. More recently, following a series of publications in 2011 [15-17], a clear international consensus pertaining to the diagnosis of first-trimester miscarriage has been established [18; see Table 9.1].

Diagnostic criteria previously varied, with guidelines being produced based on small numbers of poorly powered retrospective studies [15]. Furthermore, whilst the utility of modern TVS in the management of early pregnancy complications was becoming increasingly recognised, the reproducibility of findings was being challenged; in one study, the interobserver variation in the measurements of mean sac diameter (MSD) and crown rump length (CRL) was clinically significant (±14.64% interobserver variability) with the potential for misdiagnosis [16]. The authors recommended that any ultrasonic criterion for the diagnosis of miscarriage should take such variation into account.

Indeed, a subsequent multicentre, observational study found that the conventionally used threshold values for the diagnosis of miscarriage using CRL and MSD measurements were associated with a significant false-positive diagnosis rate for miscarriage [17]. An improved criterion for the diagnosis of miscarriage was proposed with an empty GS of MSD >25 mm, or an embryo with a CRL measurement of >7 mm without an embryonic heartbeat. Crucially these threshold values were associated with a sensitivity and positive predictive value for miscarriage of 100%. These values have now been adopted in the revised Royal College of Obstetricians and Gynaecologists (RCOG) Green-top and National Institute for Health and Care Excellence (NICE) guidance [19,20]. When measurements are around these decision boundaries or if there is any doubt about the diagnosis, then an ultrasound scan should be repeated at an interval and the ultrasound findings checked by a colleague [21]. This particularly applies where ultrasound views are compromised by the presence of fibroids, adenomyosis or an axial uterus.

Pregnancy of uncertain viability

Diagnostic difficulty arises when MSD and CRL measurements fall below the threshold values shown in Table 9.1. These pregnancies are termed 'pregnancy of uncertain viability'. Misdiagnosing a pregnancy as nonviable has serious potential implications; so, where there is any doubt, a repeat ultrasound should be arranged at an appropriate interval [18]. It should also be remembered that growth of the GS and embryo do not appear to discriminate reliably between a viable and nonviable intrauterine pregnancy of uncertain viability [22].

Predictors of miscarriage

Certain symptomatic and/or ultrasound features may increase the risk of miscarriage, e.g. heavy vaginal bleeding, or the presence of a subchorionic haematoma (Figures 9.6 and 9.7). Whilst these may aid in giving an indication as to the prognosis of the pregnancy,

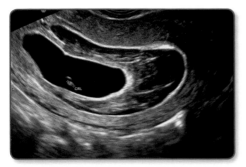

Figure 9.6 Subchorionic haematoma. There is a large crescent-shaped haematoma surrounding the gestation sac.

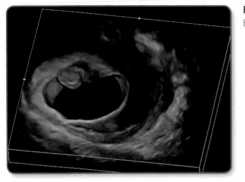

Figure 9.7 Three-dimensional image of subchorionic haematoma.

they must not be used to make a diagnosis of miscarriage. A recent study introduced a simple scoring system to predict the viability of early pregnancy <84 days using certain demographic and ultrasound features known to be predictive of miscarriage, i.e. maternal age, presence of vaginal bleeding, GS size and yolk sac size [23]. The clinical utility of such scoring systems remains unsubstantiated however.

Demographic factors

Maternal age has been found to be the most important demographic factor in miscarriage risk, particularly after 35 years of age, due to the increase in incidence of chromosomal abnormalities [8]. Increasing paternal age has also been found to play a role [8]. A history of previous pregnancy loss also increases the risk of miscarriage in subsequent pregnancies [24].

Women are most commonly referred to early pregnancy assessment units for pain and bleeding. The importance of these symptoms in determining miscarriage risk is difficult to evaluate because these symptoms are common and difficult to objectively quantify. The presence of moderate-to-heavy bleeding has, however, been shown to be associated with a higher risk of miscarriage than light bleeding [25].

Ultrasound features

When embryonic cardiac activity is visualised, the rate of subsequent miscarriage is reduced with studies showing a miscarriage rate varying from 2% to 16% [26]. The embryonic heart rate is known to progressively increase in the first trimester and bradycardia is a poor prognostic factor for pregnancy outcome at 12 weeks' gestation and should not therefore be used diagnostically [27]. A yolk sac diameter of more than two standard deviations either above or below the mean for gestation is associated with a high specificity for miscarriage [28].

The role of subchorionic haematoma as a predictor of miscarriage remains controversial. A prospective study has shown that the presence of a haematoma in the first trimester is not an independent risk factor for miscarriage after vaginal bleeding has been accounted for [29], although research is ongoing in this area.

First-trimester growth

There is increasing evidence that aberrant first-trimester growth may be associated with miscarriage. However, inaccuracies in dating pregnancies and confounding from measurements taken in pregnancies with symptoms indicative of miscarriage (i.e. pain or bleeding) have made this a complex area of study.

A link between first-trimester growth restriction and miscarriage was first highlighted in an analysis of 403 pregnancies [30]. Using customised first-trimester growth charts, the authors calculated the difference between the observed CRL of the embryos and the anticipated CRL based on the duration of amenorrhoea. The authors found that when the measured CRL lagged 7 or more days behind the expected CRL, the risk of miscarriage was significantly higher (16% vs. 5%; $P < 0.01$). Similar findings were established in a study of 292 women with spontaneously conceived singleton pregnancies with certain dates (i.e. known last menstrual period and regular menstrual cycles) presenting to an early pregnancy assessment clinic followed ultrasonically in the first trimester [31]. Although an overall trend was observed towards an overestimation of gestational age, which the authors surmised may have been a result of late ovulation, pregnancies which miscarried were found to have significantly smaller CRL. A further study used functional linear discriminant analysis (FLDA) to differentiate between embryonic growth in live pregnancies destined to miscarry, and those that continued to 14 weeks' gestation in an attempt to overcome the issue of inaccurate pregnancy dating [32]. The growth rate was derived from serial measures of CRL in the first trimester, and was compared with a single measure of CRL less than two standard deviations below that expected as a predictor of miscarriage. CRL growth rate was found to be significantly lower in the group that miscarried ($P < 0.001$). The use of FLDA was found to discriminate between normal and abnormal growth predicting miscarriage with a much higher specificity (93.1%) than a single measure of CRL (72.2%), thereby lending support to the theory of first-trimester growth restriction.

Molar pregnancy

Gestational trophoblastic disease can present as a form of miscarriage, with vaginal bleeding being the most common symptom. The gold standard for diagnosis remains histological examination of RPOC. Although rare, the classic 'snowstorm' appearance is more common with complete molar pregnancy than partial moles. Complete molar pregnancy more commonly shows a complex, intrauterine echogenic mass with cystic spaces on ultrasound scan. Partial molar pregnancies are usually seen as missed miscarriages on ultrasound and diagnosed subsequently after histological diagnosis. The accuracy of ultrasound in the diagnosis of molar pregnancy is limited. The positive predictive value has been shown to be approximately 48%, with a sensitivity of 44% [33].

Where there is ultrasound suspicion of a molar pregnancy, it is recommended that the pregnancy is managed surgically so that the diagnosis can be confirmed histologically.

MANAGEMENT OF MISCARRIAGE

The diagnosis of miscarriage can be traumatic for both the patient and partner. The couple should be given time to both absorb the diagnosis and allow management options to be comprehensively discussed. There are three options for management–expectant, medical and surgical. In the majority of cases, there is no clinical urgency to make a decision, and the patient should be given adequate opportunity to do so. Studies show that supporting a woman in her preferred method of management results in improved quality-of-life scores [34]. Many women diagnosed with miscarriage express a preference for a particular method of management which has caused difficulty in recruiting robust randomised controlled trials (RCT) in this area. The Miscarriage Treatment Trial (MIST) was an RCT specifically designed to evaluate whether there was a significant difference in infection rates between different management options. This RCT had to be prematurely concluded because of difficulties in recruitment despite being conducted in multiple centres over a period of 4 years [35].

The NICE has produced guidance in the UK which has recommended the first-line use of expectant management in women diagnosed with miscarriage unless they have a strong preference for medical or surgical treatment [20].

Expectant

Once the diagnosis of miscarriage is made, women may wait for the pregnancy to resolve spontaneously. Provided there is no evidence of infection and the woman wishes to continue with expectant management, this can continue safely for as long as is necessary. Patients are normally advised to seek medical attention if their bleeding is excessive and a routine follow-up appointment is offered to women to confirm completion of their miscarriage. The success of expectant management is dependent on the duration of follow-up and the type of miscarriage, with the highest success rates of 80-94% being associated with incomplete miscarriage. Missed miscarriage is associated with lower success rates of 28-76% for complete evacuation of the uterus [36]. NICE guidance suggests first-line expectant management for 7–14 days, although management should be individualised such that a joint decision for timescales and interventions can be made.

Medical

Medical management involves the administration of 800 µg misoprostol per vaginum to start the process of miscarriage and bleeding. This is usually offered as an outpatient procedure in the first trimester and most units in the UK now offer women the option of self-administration of vaginal misoprostol at home. This is usually followed within 2-3 hours with vaginal bleeding and pain that can be managed with simple analgesia. Women should be advised to seek medical attention if their bleeding is excessive. Oral administration is an acceptable alternative if this is the woman's preference. Sublingual misoprostol seems to have similar efficacy to oral misoprostol but with fewer side effects [37]. Guidance from the NICE suggests that women, who experience heavy bleeding which subsequently settles, do not require any further follow-up if a urine pregnancy test performed after 3 weeks is negative. In many units, however, women are asked to return after 2 weeks for repeat TVS to confirm complete miscarriage. The success rates of medical management vary widely according to the duration of follow-up and the type of miscarriage, although as with expectant management complete evacuation of the uterine cavity of products of conception is more successful with incomplete miscarriages (70-96%) than with missed miscarriages (52-92%) [38].

Surgical

Surgical management of miscarriage involves the dilatation of the cervix to allow the uterine cavity to be evacuated using suction aspiration. Success rates are high at 95-100%. In the UK, this is mainly performed under general anaesthetic; however, increasingly manual vacuum aspiration (MVA) is being used as a safe, easily performed and cost-effective outpatient alternative to traditional inpatient surgical management. The procedure is performed under local anaesthetic rather than general anaesthetic. The NICE guidance recommends the use of surgical management when expectant or medical management has failed, or when a patient has had a previous traumatic experience or is at increased risk of bleeding with nonsurgical methods.

CHOICE OF MANAGEMENT METHOD

Clinical effectiveness

It is important to be aware of the advantages and disadvantages of the different methods of management in order to better counsel women, inform shared decision making and develop an effective, patient-centred early pregnancy service.

A meta-analysis including randomised trials assigning women with first trimester missed or incomplete miscarriage to surgical, medical or expectant management showed that complete evacuation of the uterus was significantly more common with surgical than medical management (risk difference 32.8%, number needed to treat 3, success rate of medical management 62%) and with medical than expectant management (risk difference 49.7%, number needed to treat 2) [36]. Success rates with expectant management were low (39%) in comparison. It was concluded that surgical management was significantly more likely to induce complete evacuation of the uterus after miscarriage than medical management. The authors did, however, express caution in the interpretation of these findings due to the variation in quality and design of the studies included [36].

Perhaps the most well-known study to try to answer these questions was the MIST study [35]. This found the incidence of gynaecological infection after any form of management of first-trimester miscarriage to be low overall (2-3%), with little difference between the various methods. There were, however, significantly more unplanned admissions and unplanned surgical procedures after expectant and medical management than after surgical management. Often women are most concerned about the effects of these different management strategies on their future fertility. The MIST trial found that the method of miscarriage management does not affect subsequent pregnancy rates with around four in every five women giving birth within 5 years of the index miscarriage. Women can therefore be reassured that long-term fertility concerns need not affect their choice of miscarriage management.

However, economically, the MIST trial showed that expectant and medical management of first-trimester miscarriage possess significant financial advantages over surgical management [39], and the lower cost of expectant management was highlighted in a recent Cochrane review [40]. This review also found that expectant management led to a higher risk of incomplete miscarriage and need for unplanned (or additional) surgical management. In addition, the study showed higher rates of heavy bleeding and need for transfusion in women undergoing expectant management. Risk of infection and psychological outcomes were, however, similar for both groups.

Given the lack of clear superiority of any of the available approaches, the Cochrane reviews recommend that a woman's preference should be important in decision making [37]. The MIST study demonstrated that many women had a definite preference for their method of management and that women value being offered alternatives to expectant management. However, the 2012 NICE guidance recommends expectant management as first line for all women diagnosed with miscarriage (except those with a previous traumatic experience, or those at risk of heavy bleeding) [20]. This recent change in guidance has been met with considerable controversy [41] and it remains to be studied how stringently these guidelines are applied in UK early pregnancy units.

Cost-effectiveness

A cost–effectiveness study was conducted alongside the MIST trial which compared different methods of managing miscarriage taking into consideration hospital, community health and social service-related costs as well as those borne by the woman, her family and her place of employment [39]. This economic analysis showed that expectant management had clear economic advantages with the 'net societal cost' for expectant, medical and surgical management being £1086.20, £1410.10 and £1585.30 respectively. Data from the United States, however, is conflicting, showing that surgical management is more cost-effective, which may reflect the fact that this is more often performed under local anaesthetic, and therefore, with the increasing use of MVA in the UK, the financial impact may change [42].

COUNSELLING AND PSYCHOSOCIAL CONSIDERATIONS

For many couples, miscarriage is associated with significant psychological morbidity. As many as 50% of women suffer some form of psychological morbidity following a miscarriage, which may last from 6 to 12 months after the event, with a major depressive disorder reported in 10–50% of women [43]. Counselling has been shown to reduce the incidence of adverse psychological sequelae [44]. Care should emphasise a couple-centred approach. Currently, psychological support following a pregnancy loss is not offered routinely. However, in those deemed high risk, follow-up with the GP, and referral to counselling services should be considered and offered.

The importance of patient choice in the management of miscarriage may affect subsequent health-related quality of life. One study compared women who were randomised to either surgical or expectant management of miscarriage with another group of women who could not be randomised because they expressed a strong treatment preference. The study showed that women who were randomised to a particular treatment scored poorly in their subsequent quality-of-life scores compared with women who had chosen their own treatment [34].

PREVENTION OF MISCARRIAGE

The majority of miscarriages are associated with chromosomal abnormality; therefore, the prevention of miscarriages is difficult [7]. It has been suggested that some first trimester threatened miscarriages presenting with vaginal bleeding are due to suboptimal progesterone levels. Progesterone is widely used in parts of Europe in an attempt to counteract this and prevent miscarriage [45]. There is, however, little evidence to support this practice; a Cochrane review concluded that there is no evidence to support routine use of progesterone to prevent miscarriage in the first and second trimester [46]. Subgroup analysis revealed that there may be a role for progesterone in women with recurrent miscarriage. These findings were derived from the results of four small trials, three of which were published over 40 years ago, and the most recent study from 2005 was not placebo controlled. Larger trials are currently underway to inform treatment for this group of women, which includes the PRISM (Progesterone in Spontaneous Miscarriage) trial which will address the use of progesterone in women with threatened miscarriage.

It has also been suggested that women who test positive for thyroid antibodies, but have normal thyroid function, may be at increased risk of miscarriage. A RCT (TABLET) is currently underway to elucidate whether administering thyroxine to such women reduces their risk of miscarriage.

CONCLUSION

Miscarriage is a common early pregnancy condition which may be associated with significant psychological and physical morbidity. The diagnosis of miscarriage should be made according to available evidence-based guidelines. Misdiagnosis has profound implications due to the risk of terminating a desired pregnancy. Therefore, where there is diagnostic uncertainty, an expectant approach should be taken, repeating a TVS at an appropriate interval. Miscarriage may be managed expectantly, medically or surgically, and women should be provided with information about these options including success rates and complications. Women should be supported in their preference for management of miscarriage; although in the UK NICE recommends expectant management as first line treatment for most women, this approach remains controversial with many early pregnancy units supporting women in their preferred method of management. A clear treatment plan, time frame and access to emergency support and follow-up should be made available to all women irrespective of the management chosen. Psychological support in the form of support groups and counselling should be considered to prevent long-term psychological sequelae.

Key points for clinical practice

- Accuracy in diagnosing miscarriage is essential because erroneous diagnosis may result in the termination of a viable pregnancy or failure to detect an ectopic pregnancy.
- Recent consensus guidelines should be followed in the diagnosis of miscarriage, using MSD of >25 mm and CRL of >7 mm in the absence of a fetal heart in order to diagnose a miscarriage.
- Once a diagnosis is made, the options for management – expectant, medical and surgical – should be discussed and the patient supported in her choice.
- Miscarriage can be associated with significant psychological morbidity and where there are any concerns, referral to counselling services should be considered and offered.
- The aetiology of miscarriage is an interesting area of ongoing research including studies looking at the role of progesterone and thyroxine.

REFERENCES

1. Bagchi DFT. Psychological aspects of spontaneous and recurrent abortion. Curr Obstet Gynaecol 1999; 9:19–22.
2. Savitz DA, Hertz-Picciotto I, Poole C, et al. Epidemiologic measures of the course and outcome of pregnancy. Epidemiol Rev 2002; 24:91–101.
3. Condous G, Okaro E, Khalid A, et al. Do we need to follow up complete miscarriages with serum human chorionic gonadotrophin levels? BJOG 2005; 112:827–829.
4. Rulin MC, Bornstein SG, Campbell JD. The reliability of ultrasonography in the management of spontaneous abortion, clinically thought to be complete: a prospective study. Am J Obstet Gynecol 1993; 168:12–15.
5. Pandya PP, Snijders RJ, Psara N, et al. The prevalence of non-viable pregnancy at 10-13 weeks of gestation. Ultrasound Obstet Gynecol 1996; 7:170–173.
6. Casikar I, Lu C, Oates J, et al. The use of power Doppler colour scoring to predict successful expectant management in women with an incomplete miscarriage. Hum Reprod 2012; 27:669–675.
7. Ljunger E, Cnattingius S, Lundin C, et al. Chromosomal anomalies in first-trimester miscarriages. Acta Obstet Gynecol Scand 2005; 84:1103–1107.
8. de la Rochebrochard E, Thonneau P. Paternal age and maternal age are risk factors for miscarriage; results of a multicentre European study. Hum Reprod 2002; 17:1649–1656.
9. Backos M, Rai R, Baxter N, et al. Pregnancy complications in women with recurrent miscarriage associated with antiphospholipid antibodies treated with low dose aspirin and heparin. Br J Obstet Gynaecol 1999; 106:102–107.
10. Hawthorne G, Robson S, Ryall EA, et al. Prospective population based survey of outcome of pregnancy in diabetic women: results of the Northern Diabetic Pregnancy Audit, 1994. BMJ 1997; 315:279–281.
11. Cocksedge KA, Li TC, Saravelos SH, et al. A reappraisal of the role of polycystic ovary syndrome in recurrent miscarriage. Reprod Biomed Online 2008; 17:151–160.
12. Pineles BL, Park E, Samet JM. Systematic review and meta-analysis of miscarriage and maternal exposure to tobacco smoke during pregnancy. Am J Epidemiol 2014; 179:807–823.
13. Jayaprakasan K, Chan YY, Sur S, et al. Prevalence of uterine anomalies and their impact on early pregnancy in women conceiving after assisted reproduction treatment. Ultrasound Obstet Gynecol 2011; 37:727–732.
14. Goldstein SR. Early Pregnancy: Normal and abnormal. Semin Reprod Med 2008; 26:277–283.
15. Jeve Y, Rana R, Bhide A, et al. Accuracy of first-trimester ultrasound in the diagnosis of early embryonic demise: a systematic review. Ultrasound Obstet Gynecol 2011; 38:489–496.
16. Pexsters A, Luts J, Van Schoubroeck D, et al. Clinical implications of intra- and interobserver reproducibility of transvaginal sonographic measurement of gestational sac and crown-rump length at 6-9 weeks' gestation. Ultrasound Obstet Gynecol 2011; 38:510–515.
17. Abdallah Y, Daemen A, Kirk E, et al. Limitations of current definitions of miscarriage using mean gestational sac diameter and crown-rump length measurements: a multicenter observational study. Ultrasound Obstet Gynecol 2011; 38:497–502.
18. Doubilet PM, Benson CB, Bourne T, et al. Diagnostic criteria for nonviable pregnancy early in the first trimester. N Engl J Med 2013; 369:1443–1451.
19. Royal College of Obstetricians & Gynaecologists (RCOG). Early pregnancy loss, management (green-top guideline no. 25). London; RCOG, 2006:1–18.
20. National Institute for Health and Care Excellence (NICE). Ectopic pregnancy and miscarriage: diagnosis and initial management in early ectopic pregnancy and miscarriage. CG154. London; NICE, 2012.
21. Bourne T, Bottomley C. When is a pregnancy nonviable and what criteria should be used to define miscarriage? Fertil Steril 2012; 98:1091–1096.
22. Abdallah Y, Daemen A, Guha S, et al. Gestational sac and embryonic growth are not useful as criteria to define miscarriage: a multicenter observational study. Ultrasound Obstet Gynecol 2011; 38:503–509.
23. Bottomley C, Van Belle V, Kirk E, et al. Accurate prediction of pregnancy viability by means of a simple scoring system. Hum Reprod 2013; 28:68–76.
24. Maconochie N, Doyle P, Prior S, et al. Risk factors for first trimester miscarriage—results from a UK-population-based case-control study. BJOG 2007; 114:170–186.
25. Poulose T, Richardson R, Ewings P, et al. Probability of early pregnancy loss in women with vaginal bleeding and a singleton live fetus at ultrasound scan. J Obstet Gynaecol 2006; 26:782–784.

26. Makrydimas G, Sebire NJ, Lolis D, et al. Fetal loss following ultrasound diagnosis of a live fetus at 6-10 weeks of gestation. Ultrasound Obstet Gynecol 2003; 22:368–372.
27. Makrydimas G, Papanikolaou E, Paraskevaidis E, et al. Upper limb abnormalities as an isolated ultrasonographic finding in early detection of trisomy 18. A case report. Fetal Diagn Ther 2003; 18:401–403.
28. Küçük T, Duru N, Yenen M, et al. Yolk sac size and shape as predictors of poor pregnancy outcome. J Perinat Med 1999; 27:316–320.
29. Johns J, Hyett J, Jauniaux E. Obstetric outcome after threatened miscarriage with and without a hematoma on ultrasound. Obstet Gynecol 2003; 102:483–487.
30. Koornstra G, Wattel E, Exalto N. Crown-rump length measurements revisited. Eur J Obstet Gynecol Reprod Biol 1990; 35:131–130.
31. Mukri F, Bourne T, Bottomley C, et al. Evidence of early first-trimester growth restriction in pregnancies that subsequently end in miscarriage. BJOG 2008; 115:1273–1278.
32. Bottomley C, Daemen A, Mukri F, et al. Functional linear discriminant analysis: a new longitudinal approach to the assessment of embryonic growth. Hum Reprod 2009; 24:278–283.
33. Kirk E, Papageorghiou AT, Condous G, et al. The accuracy of first trimester ultrasound in the diagnosis of hydatidiform mole. Ultrasound Obstet Gynecol 2007; 29:70–75.
34. Wieringa-De Waard M, Hartman E, Ankum W, et al. Expectant management versus surgical evacuation in first trimester miscarriage: health-related quality of life in randomized and non-randomized patients. Hum Reprod 2002; 17:1638–1642.
35. Trinder J, Brocklehurst P, Porter R, et al. Management of miscarriage: expectant, medical, or surgical? Results of randomised controlled trial (miscarriage treatment (MIST) trial). BMJ 2006; 332:1235–1240.
36. Sotiriadis A, Makrydimas G, Papatheodorou S, et al. Expectant, medical, or surgical management of first-trimester miscarriage: a meta-analysis. Obstet Gynecol 2005; 105:1104–1113.
37. von Hertzen H, Huong NT, Piaggio G, et al. Misoprostol dose and route after mifepristone for early medical abortion: a randomised controlled noninferiority trial. BJOG 2010; 117:1186–1196.
38. Neilson JP, Gyte GM, Hickey M, et al. Medical treatments for incomplete miscarriage. Cochrane Database Syst Rev 2013; 3:CD007223.
39. Petrou S, Trinder J, Brocklehurst P, et al. Economic evaluation of alternative management methods of first-trimester miscarriage based on results from the MIST trial. BJOG 2006; 113:879–889.
40. Nanda K, Lopez LM, Grimes DA, et al. Expectant care versus surgical treatment for miscarriage. Cochrane Database Syst Rev 2012; 3:CD003518.
41. Bourne T, Barnhart K, Benson CB, et al. NICE guidance on ectopic pregnancy and miscarriage restricts access and choice and may be clinically unsafe. BMJ 2013; 346:f197.
42. Sagili H, Divers M. Economic evaluation of alternative management methods of first-trimester miscarriage based on results from the miscarriage treatment (MIST) trial by Petrou et al. BJOG 2007; 114:116–117.
43. Lok IH, Neugebauer R. Psychological morbidity following miscarriage. Best Pract Res Clin Obstet Gynaecol 2007; 21:229–247.
44. Swanson K. Effects of caring, measurement, and time on miscarriage impact and women's well-being. Nurs Res 1999; 48:288–298.
45. Beyens MN, Guy C, Ratrema M, et al. Prescription of drugs to pregnant women in France: the HIMAGE study. Therapie 2003; 58:505–511.
46. Haas DM, Ramsey PS. Progestogen for preventing miscarriage. Cochrane Database Syst Rev 2013; 10:CD003511.

Chapter 10

The future of cervical screening

Nirmala Rai, David Luesley

INTRODUCTION

Cervical screening has come a long way since the advent of the Papanicolaou smear in the 1940s. The introduction of cervical screening of women to prevent cervical cancer, by identifying and treating precancerous cells, has had its share of proponents and detractors. Cervical screening initially met with both criticism and scepticism [1–3] before gaining widespread acceptance in the late 20th century. The evolution of cervical screening from an ad hoc investigation into organised national screening programmes has led to significant reductions in the incidence of cervical cancer in the developed world.

The identification of oncogenic human papilloma viruses (HPV) as the underlying causes of cervical cancer has led to the development of prophylactic HPV vaccines; vaccination of pre-teenage and teenage children against HPV 16 and 18 is now common in many parts of the developed world. The recognition of HPVs' prime aetiological role in cervical disease has also changed the cervical screening programme from a primarily cytological based process to an HPV-based one, with HPV tests now being employed for both triage and test of cure. Despite these advances, cervical cancers remain highly prevalent in the developing world with corresponding high rates of mortality.

CURRENT CERVICAL SCREENING IN DEVELOPED COUNTRIES

Developed countries have been able to implement effective cervical screening programmes that have significantly reduced both the incidence and mortality from cervical cancer. There is evidence suggesting that deaths from cervical cancer can be reduced by 95% if 80% of the eligible 25- to 64-year-old female population is covered. In 2010/11 the coverage of eligible women in the UK was 78.6%.

The cervical screening programme in the UK might be regarded as a model of a successful screening programme in the developed world. Women are invited to have a cervical smear between the ages of 25 and 64 years. The test is undertaken on a 3-yearly basis until the age of 49 and 5-yearly until the age of 64. Only women with previous

Nirmala Rai MBBS MRCOG, Cancer sciences, University of Birmingham, Birmingham, UK. Email: nimarai18@doctors. org.uk (for correspondence)

David Luesley MA MD FRCOG, Gyn Oncology, Sandwell and West Birmingham Hospitals, Birmingham, UK

abnormal smears or women who have never been screened before 50 years of age are invited for further cervical screening beyond the age of 65 years.

The National Health Service Cervical Screening Programme (NHSCSP) changed from conventional cytology to liquid-based cytology (LBC) in 2008. LBC is more efficient with a reduced incidence of inadequate smears, quicker turnover time and the added advantage of 'reflex' HPV testing. Reflex high-risk (HR) HPV testing is done when the cervical smear results are inconclusive [i.e. borderline or atypical squamous cells of undetermined significance (ASCUS)] and helps to triage women into those who need further testing with colposcopy (test positive) and those who can return to routine screening (test negative). In 2012, HPV testing HR types was introduced to triage women with abnormal (borderline or low grade) smears and to provide a test of cure with the aim of further improving clinical outcomes and screening efficiency after successful implementation of the HPV sentinel sites project in 2008 [4].

HPV testing has been shown to have greater sensitivity (+37%) but lower specificity (−7%) for cervical intraepithelial neoplasia (CIN)2 or worse (high-grade squamous intraepithelial lesions or HSIL) compared with cytology [5]. Testing for HPV is also more reproducible than cytology using a cut-point of mild dyskaryosis or less (low-grade squamous intraepithelial lesions or LSIL) [5]. In a meta-analysis, the pooled sensitivity with HPV DNA testing was significantly higher than cytology to detect high-grade lesions (CIN2 and CIN3) in ASCUS/borderline triage with similar pooled sensitivity. Contrary to earlier expectations, HPV testing was not equally effective for triage of LSIL/mild abnormal cytology as the pooled specificity was shown to be significantly lower, even though the pooled sensitivity is higher [6].

Women who have been treated for high-grade lesions are between two and five times more likely to develop cervical cancer [7,8] and over 50% of these cancers occur in women who are lost to follow-up or in women who do not engage in cervical screening [9]. Women who are HPV-negative are at very low risk of developing subsequent disease. Following treatment, women who have borderline changes or mild dyskaryosis in smears at 6 months are tested for HPV. HPV-negative women are recalled for a repeat test only after 3 years, and hence avoid annual screening for 10 years as per previous protocols. Women who are either HPV test positive or have high-grade abnormalities (i.e. moderate or severe dyskaryosis) are returned to colposcopy. This strategy is termed 'Test of Cure'. Eighty per cent of women following treatment are expected to be returned to routine screening following HPV test of cure. Combined testing with HPV and cytology was noted to be equally sensitive to HPV testing but significantly less specific [6]. Pooled sensitivity (meta-analysis) for HPV testing post-treatment was more sensitive (93%) in comparison to cytology (72%), but equally specific (81% vs. 84%), thus safely allowing the use of HPV testing as test of cure [6].

EFFECT OF VACCINATION ON CERVICAL SCREENING

The HPV vaccine (both bivalent and quadrivalent) will protect against high-grade HPV types 16 and 18 which are responsible for 80% of cervical cancers. The effect of vaccine is projected to have little impact on cervical cancer burden until another 10 years, although there will be an effect on the types and prevalence of abnormal cervical smears. Some cross-immunity is expected, but it is logical to expect that HPV vaccination will not protect against other HR HPV strains which have the potential to cause dyskaryosis and neoplasia.

Early data on the effect of vaccination indicate that high-grade abnormalities are significantly reduced in vaccinated women, but the incidence of low-grade abnormalities remains largely unchanged [10]. The impact of vaccination in the UK is predicted to result in a 10% overall decrease in abnormal cytology; 50% decrease in high-grade CIN and a 70% decrease in cervical cancer [11]. There will be no changes in the groups who were not vaccinated because of their age at the time of the inception of the vaccination programme.

Colposcopy is more sensitive than cytology in detecting high-grade abnormalities, but it is less specific and likely to be biased by prior knowledge of the cytology results [11]. The positive predictive value (PPV) of cytology is expected to decrease as a result of the lower prevalence of cytological changes in the screened population. In addition, there may be a direct effect on the performance of cytoscreeners caused by reduced exposure to abnormal cells and pattern recognition. Reduction in the PPV of cytology may also influence colposcopy. False-positive cytology results are likely to increase the number of women referred for colposcopy with the potential for unnecessary intervention and causing additional anxiety in those women referred. Whilst these are potential adverse outcomes, it is still early days and further evidence is awaited on the effect of HPV immunisation on the performance of cytology and colposcopy within cervical screening.

PRIMARY SCREENING WITH HPV

Since screening began, it has relied upon the morphological interpretation of the exfoliated cells in smears. Organised cervical screening programmes have reduced cervical cancer-related mortality by nearly 50%. Cytology standards are influenced by the quality of samples, interpretation of morphological changes in cells, which can be subjective and influenced by interpretive errors. An understanding that HPV infection is a necessary prerequisite in the genesis of cervical cancer has allowed for new developments in both detection and possible prevention. This knowledge and understanding has made it possible for a new effective primary prevention with vaccination and caused a significant shift from a morphological to a virological basis for secondary prevention.

There are many studies that suggest that HPV-based primary screening has better sensitivity. Women who are screened HPV-negative have a greatly reduced risk of cancer, and as the latent period from infection to affliction is long we will be able to safely increase the interval between screenings. Apart from providing greater sensitivity, they are also unaffected by subjective observations. When compared to cytology, the main limitation of primary HPV screening is its reduced specificity, especially in women younger than 35 years due to a higher prevalence of transient infections [12]. It is possible that this limitation may be partially offset by the reduced PPV of cytology predicted in the future [13]. Primary screening based upon HPV would facilitate creating a registry of HPV prevalence and may be used to monitor the epidemiology of HPV infection and the effect of vaccination in the population.

The International Agency for Research on Cancer issued a statement in 2005 concluding that HPV testing is at least as effective as cytology [14]. The NHSCSP is currently piloting HPV primary screening in the UK which was rolled out in 2013 in six pilot centres. The results are awaited before an HPV-based screening programme is designed and new screening algorithms are put in place. The United States (US) Food and Drug Administration (FDA) announced approval for HPV test for first-line HPV primary screening in the United States in April 2014 in women aged over 25. This HPV screening

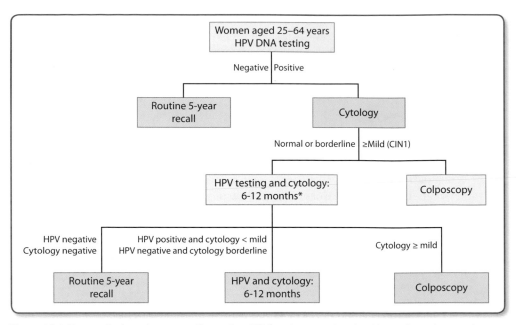

Figure 10.1 Proposed primary human papilloma virus (HPV) testing screening algorithm with cytology used to triage HPV-positive women. Adapted from Cuzick et al 2008 [25]. *An alternative to using HPV and cytology testing at 2nd round would be to apply HPV 16 testing to triage women who are HPV and cytology positive for borderline or mildly abnormal dyskaryotic cells..

strategy tests for 14 HR HPV types, and women who test positive for HPV 16 and 18 are immediately referred for colposcopy. Women testing positive for other HR HPV types are tested with cytology to triage referral to colposcopy.

Current models of primary HPV testing using cytological triage, combining the high specificity of cytology with the higher sensitivity of HPV testing, have demonstrated greater effectiveness [15,16]. The more sensitive HPV testing is applied first followed by cytology. Women who are HPV-positive but cytology-negative can be safely managed by repeating both the tests after 12 months, and referring women with positive results (abnormal cytology) to colposcopy and returning double negative results, negative HPV and cytology to routine screening [17,18]. A flow chart showing a potential management algorithm based upon primary screening with HPV is given in **Figure 10.1**.

A negative HR HPV test provides better protection against CIN ≥ 2, ≥CIN3 and cervical cancer than cytology as shown in several longitudinal studies [18–20]. It may be possible to extend the screening interval to 6 or even 8 years (especially in women who are HPV-negative) without increasing the lifetime cancer risk [21] when primary HR HPV screening is introduced. Another HPV-based screening guideline incorporates the impact of vaccination and the longer safety interval in HPV-negative women [22]:

• Vaccinated women between ages 11 and 14 years could be screened just twice at the ages of 30 and 45.
• Vaccinated women between ages 15 and 23 years could be screened once at the age of 25, and then twice more at 35 and 50. Women who are already sexually active prior to vaccination are less protected and hence a first screen at 25 is useful to detect women not protected by the vaccine.

- Unvaccinated women (or who have not completed all three doses) should be screened more regularly at the ages of 25, 30, 35, 45 and 55 years.

Several triage screening strategies have been suggested based upon results from different clinical trials, but to date the optimal approach in terms of clinical outcomes is still to be elucidated [21].

The current cervical screening programme places a large economic burden on the health sector in its present format. Simply reducing the frequency of cervical screening may not be a solution because it may affect cytological and clinical quality standards. It is essential that the current programme evolves in keeping with the advances in basic science. However, adaptions to screening protocols should be introduced carefully within organised programmes as part of an evolving process with evaluation of clinical outcomes so that the success of current programmes is not compromised.

PREVENTING CERVICAL CANCER IN RESOURCE-POOR COUNTRIES

The bulk of cervical cancer (80%) occurs in resource-poor countries and is the leading cause of death from cancer in women in the developing world [23]. Only 5% of women in the developing world are estimated to undergo screening in comparison to 50% in the developed world [24]. There are a multitude of reasons why cervical disease is more common in resource-poor countries and why there is an apparent lack of progress in combating cervical cancer in the developing world. Reasons include the absence of an organised screening programme, the lack of awareness amongst women and care providers compounded by inadequate training, limited financial resources, restricted access to medical care, poor quality of cytological and colposcopy services and a lack of political will. Primary testing for HPV has helped overcome some of the challenges and obstacles associated with implementing conventional cytology-based screening programmes. The need for multiple clinic visits required with conventional programmes formulated in the developed world is not sustainable in the developing world. A quick, low cost, low technology method of screening, diagnosis and treatment is essential for screening to be effective in these settings. Studies of visual inspection of the cervix after application of acetic acid (VIA) or Lugol's iodine (VILI) and HPV testing as stand-alone or in tandem have shown promising results as efficient alternatives [25].

VIA/VILI is an inexpensive screening method and the consumable solutions are widely available. A 'see and treat' approach can be employed as both methods yield immediate results and a large number of personnel including nurses and paramedical staff can be trained quickly [26]. The pooled sensitivity of VIA varies from 62% to 80% and the specificity from 77% to 84% in the detection of high-grade lesions, after adjusting for verification bias [27]. VILI has comparable accuracy to studies reporting VIA; a multicentre study conducted in India and Africa showed a pooled sensitivity and specificity of 77% and 86% respectively for VIA versus 92% and 85% for VILI. However, estimates of sensitivity were significantly lower (53%) for detecting high-grade lesions (CIN $\geq$2) by VILI in another study conducted in Latin America [28,29]. In a further trial conducted in rural India, women were tested for HPV, cytology or VIA, with appropriate treatment of precancerous lesions and cervical cancer. A single round of HPV testing was reported to be associated with a significant reduction in the numbers of advanced cervical cancers (FIGO stage 2+) and cervical cancer-related deaths [30].

Prevention of cervical cancer requires two co-ordinated activities – timely, accurate screening followed by effective early treatment of preinvasive lesions. Cryotherapy for treatment is reported to be easier to perform, which is safe, effective and an acceptable method of treatment in resource-poor settings and has reported cure rates of 81.4% for CIN1, 71.4% for CIN2 and 68% for CIN3 [31]. Cryotherapy is less expensive and easier to perform when compared to large loop excision of the transformation zone. Another rural Indian study showed the test positive rates to be 14% for VIA, 7% for cytology and 10.3% for the 'screen and treat' approach (cryotherapy following either HPV or VIA +ve) [32], a strategy that has been shown to be more effective when compared to delayed treatment for high grade lesions in unscreened women aged 35–65 years [33]. An HPV DNA test (CareHPV Qiagen, Gaithersburg) has been developed recently specifically for women in low-resource settings. It detects 14 HR types of HPV in about 2.5 hours, thus allowing rapid testing and clinical follow-up on the same day, enabling a more efficient single setting screening and treatment based upon primary HPV testing.

The clinical accuracy of CareHPV as a rapid screening test was evaluated on both operator-obtained cervical specimens and patient-obtained vaginal specimens in a cross-sectional study in rural China. The sensitivity and specificity of the CareHPV test for a cut-off ratio cut-point of 0.5 relative units were 90 and 84.2% respectively on cervical specimens and 81.4% and 82.4% on vaginal specimens. The overall accuracy between screening tests, as summarised by the relative areas under a receiver operating curve, was not significantly different. The area under the curve also did not differ significantly when compared to hybrid capture 2 (HC2)--an HPV DNA test that tests for 13 HPV HR types and the first HPV test approved by the FDA but was significantly better in comparison to VIA (41.4% and 94.5%) to detect high-grade lesions. Combining HPV and/or VIA testing with the immediate treatment of women who are test positive has many advantages, and a possible algorithm is proposed in **Figure 10.2**. One of the limitations of HPV testing is the low specificity and in the absence of a good supporting colposcopy services one must be mindful of the potential to overtreat a large number of women who have transient infections or low-grade/no cervical disease. More studies are needed to carefully evaluate the advantage of treating potential precancerous lesions offset by the side effects experienced by women without cervical disease.

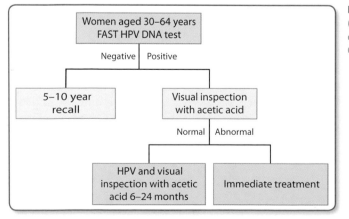

Figure 10.2 Human papillomavirus (HPV) based screening proposed for developing countries. Adapted from Cuzick J et al. 2008 [25].

A two-dose prophylactic HPV vaccine has now also been made available to the developing world by Global Alliance for Vaccines and Immunization (GAVI) alliance at a lower cost of £2.90 per dose, which potentially could see more widespread use in impoverished countries with a consequent reduction in mortality from cervical cancer [34].

COULD SELF-TESTING BECOME THE STANDARD?

Many patients referred to colposcopy do not attend either diagnosis, treatment or follow-up. Nonattendance of women may be due to procedure-related anxiety, embarrassment, inconvenience, fear of medical personnel or pain, lack of time or forgetting appointments. In resource-poor settings, the additional problems of scarcity of trained personnel and adequate infrastructure limit comprehensive service provision further. The changing paradigm with a shift from cytology-based testing towards HPV screening offers opportunities to explore alternative methods of specimen collection such as vaginal collection of samples that obviates the need for an uncomfortable speculum examination and may improve patient compliance and screening coverage.

Vaginal collection of samples also extends the possibility for the collection to be operator independent, i.e. self-collection by women. Studies have shown that HPV testing done on vaginal specimens is as accurate as samples collected from the cervix; Finan et al collected samples from the vagina by Ayres spatula and found 100% concordance with cervical samples [35]. In contrast, other studies have reported discordance and variable sensitivity for HPV detection in vaginal samples when compared to cervical samples, although the variance observed may be due to different collection methods, sampling techniques, operator (self vs. trained personnel) or timing of the two samples [36,37]. A systematic review and meta-analysis, examining self-sampling versus physician-collected cervical samples not only showed good patient acceptance, but also reported that self-sampling was preferred by the majority of women. The review concluded that self-sampling was as sensitive as physician-obtained samples to detect HPV DNA or HR HPV DNA, but noted a wide heterogeneity between different studies. A study conducted in Sweden using a novel self-sampling device also showed high patient acceptance and good concordance of HPV results between self-collected and clinician-collected samples [38].

Fifty percent of cervical cancers occur in women who are noncompliant with cervical screening, and self-sampling removes some of the obstacles posed by current sampling techniques and may be a way forward for many women who are likely to default [39]. A degree of caution may need to be exercised in the initial interpretation of the results of HPV vaccination programme. Encouraging results with reduced case load in the beginning may potentially represent vaccinated women who historically may have shown high screening compliance, as they reflect women who are already well motivated and have good awareness and unlikely to have developed cervical cancer, whereas nonattenders may harbour lesions that progress undetected and present at a later date as cervical cancer [13]. Apart from being an attractive option in nonattenders, self-sampling is also less expensive, less invasive, better tolerated by women and may be more convenient. HPV DNA remains relatively stable over time and can easily be transported to distant centres, allowing for a more robust central infrastructure [40]. Hence, it could also be used in low-resource settings. Currently, there is no consensus on the best sampling procedure. However, accumulating evidence appears to support self-sampling [41].

THE MOLECULAR FUTURE

One of the main limitations of HPV testing is its poor specificity in comparison to cytology. This may result in increased referral to colposcopy services and possible overtreatment. Advances in HPV testing have led to the discovery of promising biomarkers based on the understanding of the natural history of HPV-dependent cervical carcinogenesis. Biomarkers appear to have increased specificity when compared to HPV DNA testing alone and may have roles in improving triage (i.e. recommend colposcopy, instigate treatment, undertake intensive monitoring or discharge) in HR HPV-positive women. By reducing false-positive diagnoses, unnecessary treatment or surveillance may be minimised. HPV genotyping, viral load analysis, E6/E7 expression analysis, p16INK4a (p16), Ki-67 and promoter methylation analysis of tumour suppressor genes are some of the biomarkers that have been studied and show promise.

HR HPV E6 and E7 oncoproteins interact with p53 and pRB respectively and are expressed heavily in the basal and parabasal cells of high-grade CIN. Overexpression of E6 and E7 genes in the integrated HPV genome is necessary for progression to malignancy and indicates a shift from the productive phase to transformative phase of HPV infection. Testing for high levels on E6/E7 mRNA in cervical smears provides a higher specificity and higher predictive value for high-grade lesions than the DNA assays and may serve as a superior triage tool by enhancing prediction of progressive disease [42]. In another study, it was noted that mRNA positivity increased with the severity of the cervical lesions and women with ≥CIN2 were more likely to test positive with mRNA testing. Thus, mRNA testing (using PreTect HPV-proofer) may be of value in triaging women with HR HPV DNA-positive and normal cytology for colposcopy [43]. Testing with mRNA appears to be potentially more efficient than cytology for the triage of HPV DNA-positive women [44].

Viral load analysis may also predict progression of CIN ≥ 2 lesions and may be more useful in low-resource settings with poor cytology triage [45]. HPV 16 and 18 cause 70% of cervical cancers, and a supplementary genotyping assay to detect HR HPV 16 and 18 can be used as a triage for immediate referral to colposcopy. Cyclin-dependent kinase inhibitor p16 is another biomarker that is upregulated either alone or in combination and has improved sensitivity to detect high-grade lesions. It has been suggested that p16 is a useful marker to detect CIN ≥ 2 lesions, especially in cases with cytohistological discordance because of its higher accuracy for ASCUS and LSIL after triage with HR HPV tests [46]. A systematic review and meta-analysis on p16 immunocytochemistry versus HPV testing for triage of women with minor cytological abnormalities confirms the improved accuracy of p16 in comparison to HC2 testing for triage of women with ASCUS and LSIL, but showed less sensitivity for LSIL triage [47]. Heterogeneity in results has been noted between morphological and quantitative studies and a new dual immunostain (CINtec plus) may help to simplify the test [48]. Ki-67 is regarded as a surrogate marker for deregulated cell proliferation, and combined testing for both p16 and Ki-67 has been reported to have a high sensitivity and specificity of 91.9 and 82.1% for detection of CIN ≥ 2 and 96.4% and 76.9% for CIN3+ respectively [48].

CADM1 and MAL are tumour suppressor genes that may also be useful biomarkers, where supermethylation of the promoter region can be detected on a methylation marker panel. It has been shown to be at least equally discriminatory for high-grade CIN (CIN2 and CIN3) as cytology in HR HPV-positive women, or as cytology with the detection of

HPV16/18. It has been demonstrated that the methylation levels of the two genes reflect the increasing severity and duration of the cervical disease and markedly increased levels are seen in cervical cancer. Biomarker assays are promising developments and also have the advantage of providing more objectivity than cytology. There remains considerable heterogeneity between different studies; thus larger, longitudinal studies in target populations are needed to confirm clinical utility. There are also other biomarkers of interest under investigation such as gain of 3q chromosomal abnormality, short coding RNAs (miRNA), proteomics, markers of aberrant S-phase induction [topoisomerase IIA and mini-chromosome maintenance protein 2 (MCM2)], cellular makers such as CK13 and CK14, MCM5 and CDC6 and Survivin which also have shown promise in small studies.

IMPACT OF HPV-BASED SCREENING ON INFRASTRUCTURE

HPV is being used as a triage tool for low-grade cervical smears, especially for ASCUS and for test of cure. Some countries have changed from cytology to HPV-based primary screening, and the results from pilot studies are awaited in other countries including the UK. The main limitation of shifting to a screening programme based on HPV primary screening is the poor specificity of HPV in those <35 years of age and especially women <30 years because of the high prevalence of transient infections. This may lead to an increase in colposcopy referrals and possible overtreatment of women. In addition, there is concern over a possible decline in the negative predictive value of cytology. However, these concerns may be eased if the emerging research showing the potential utility of biomarkers to improve specificity of screening is realised. The future screening programme may then become entirely HPV based using biomarkers for secondary testing or using cytology as triage tool.

The financial burden on the system is also a growing concern in developed countries. This burden will be potentially reduced by the safe extension of screening duration in HPV-negative women. HPV testing requires no specialised tools and many tests can be run from a single laboratory platform; the simplified laboratory test allows good quality assurance, as it is objective. Testing can also be centralised. In the developing world where there is no organised screening programme, there is potential benefit from a centralised HPV-based programme or from rapid HPV testing that allows for screen and treat services where all interventions are undertaken at the same visit. Screening recommendations may vary in different regions of the world as risk thresholds and available resources differ substantially; the relative risks versus benefits within the local population will need to be considered to formulate and introduce appropriate programmes.

CONCLUSION

Preventing cervical cancer through cervical screening remains a high priority health objective. Advances in health technologies have provided interventions such as HPV vaccination and have driven the paradigm shift from cytology-based towards HPV-based testing. With increased understanding of the natural history of cervical disease, advances in basic science and development of new diagnostic tests, it is essential to re-examine and re-evaluate existing screening practices to optimise safety, acceptability and cost-effectiveness.

Key points for clinical practice

- High risk oncogenic HPV is an essential cause of cervical cancer.
- HPV 16 and 18 cause 70% of cervical cancer.
- Bivalent (HPV 16 and 18) and quadrivalent (HPV 6, 11, 16 and 18) prophylactic vaccines are currently available as primary prevention.
- HPV vaccination does not eliminate the need for routine cervical screening.
- A paradigm shift from cytology towards HPV testing is being seen in cervical screening.
- Reduced specificity and transient HPV infection in women younger than 30 is one of the challenging limitations of HPV testing.
- Advances in HPV testing have led to discovery and development of biomarkers assays with potential to improve HPV testing further in future.
- Introduction of primary HPV testing with increased duration between screening for HPV-negative women and self-testing in nonattenders could all be potential future developments.
- A large burden of mortality from cervical cancer remains in resource-poor countries which may improve with CareHPV testing and other strategies that reduce dependence on cytology (as cytology-based screening is iterative, needs expertise and is expensive).

REFERENCES

1. Cochrane AL. Effectiveness and efficiency: random reflections on health services. London: The Nuffield Hospitals Trust, 1972.
2. Lund CJ. An epitaph for cervical carcinoma. JAMA 1961; 175:98–99.
3. Saffron L. Cervical cancer: the politics of prevention. Spare Rib 1983; 129:47.
4. Moss SKR, Legood R, Sadique Z, et al. Evaluation of sentinel sites for HPV triage and test of cure2011. Available from: http://www.cancerscreening.nhs.uk/cervical/sentinelfinalreport.pdf.
5. Arbyn M, Sasieni P, Meijer CJ, et al. Clinical applications of HPV testing: a summary of meta-analyses. Vaccine 2006; 24 (Suppl 3):S3/78–89.
6. Arbyn M, Ronco G, Anttila A, et al. Evidence regarding human papillomavirus testing in secondary prevention of cervical cancer. Vaccine 2012; 30 (Suppl 5):F88–F99.
7. Soutter WP, de Barros Lopes A, Fletcher A, et al. Invasive cervical cancer after conservative therapy for cervical intraepithelial neoplasia. Lancet 1997; 349:978–980.
8. Strander B, Andersson-Ellstrom A, Milsom I, et al. Long term risk of invasive cancer after treatment for cervical intraepithelial neoplasia grade 3: population based cohort study. BMJ 2007; 335:1077.
9. Soutter WP, Sasieni P, Panoskaltsis T. Long-term risk of invasive cervical cancer after treatment of squamous cervical intraepithelial neoplasia. Int J Cancer 2006; 118:2048–2055.
10. Brotherton JM, Fridman M, May CL, et al. Early effect of the HPV vaccination programme on cervical abnormalities in Victoria, Australia: an ecological study. Lancet 2011; 377:2085–2092.
11. The implications of HPV vaccinations for colposcopy: BSCCP; 2013. Available from: https://www.bsccp.org.uk/healthcare-professionals/professional-news/the-implications-of-hpv-vaccinations-for-colposcopy/.
12. Cuzick J, Clavel C, Petry KU, et al. Overview of the European and North American studies on HPV testing in primary cervical cancer screening. Int J Cancer 2006; 119:1095–1101.
13. Franco EL, Cuzick J, Hildesheim A, et al. Issues in planning cervical cancer screening in the era of HPV vaccination. Vaccine 2006; 24 (Suppl 3):S3/171–177.
14. IARC. Handbooks of cancer prevention, vol 10. Cervix cancer screening. Lyon: IARC Press; 2005.
15. Ronco G, Giorgi-Rossi P, Carozzi F, et al. Efficacy of human papillomavirus testing for the detection of invasive cervical cancers and cervical intraepithelial neoplasia: a randomised controlled trial. Lancet Oncol 2010; 11:249–257.
16. Zorzi M, Del Mistro A, Farruggio A, et al. Use of a high-risk human papillomavirus DNA test as the primary test in a cervical cancer screening programme: a population-based cohort study. BJOG 2013; 120:1260-1267; discussion 7–8.

17. Cuzick J, Szarewski A, Cubie H, et al. Management of women who test positive for high-risk types of human papillomavirus: the HART study. Lancet 2003; 362:1871–1876.
18. Rijkaart DC, Berkhof J, Rozendaal L, et al. Human papillomavirus testing for the detection of high-grade cervical intraepithelial neoplasia and cancer: final results of the POBASCAM randomised controlled trial. Lancet Oncol 2012; 13:78–88.
19. Dillner J, Rebolj M, Birembaut P, et al. Long term predictive values of cytology and human papillomavirus testing in cervical cancer screening: Joint European Cohort Study. BMJ 2008; 337:a1754.
20. Ronco G, Dillner J, Elfstrom KM, et al. Efficacy of HPV-based screening for prevention of invasive cervical cancer: follow-up of four European randomised controlled trials. Lancet 2014; 383:524–532.
21. Dijkstra MG, Snijders PJ, Arbyn M, et al. Cervical cancer screening: on the way to a shift from cytology to full molecular screening. Ann Oncol 2014; 25:927–935.
22. Young E. Cancer Research UK. 2010. Available from: NCRI conference: How could the HPV vaccine change cervical screening.
23. GLOBOCAN 2012: Estimated Cancer Incidence, Mortality and Prevalence Worldwide in 2012 [Internet]. International Agency for Research on Cancer. 2012. Available from: http://globocan.iarc.fr.2012.
24. Control of cancer of the cervix uteri. A WHO Meeting. Bull World Health Organ 1986; 64:607–618.
25. Cuzick J, Arbyn M, Sankaranarayanan R, et al. Overview of human papillomavirus-based and other novel options for cervical cancer screening in developed and developing countries. Vaccine 2008; 26 (Suppl 10):K29–K41.
26. Blumenthal PD, Lauterbach M, Sellors JW, et al. Training for cervical cancer prevention programs in low-resource settings: focus on visual inspection with acetic acid and cryotherapy. Int J Gynaecol Obstet 2005; 89 (Suppl 2):S30–S37.
27. Sankaranarayanan R, Gaffikin L, Jacob M, et al. A critical assessment of screening methods for cervical neoplasia. Int J Gynaecol Obstet 2005; 89 (Suppl 2):S4–S12.
28. Sankaranarayanan R, Basu P, Wesley RS, et al. Accuracy of visual screening for cervical neoplasia: results from an IARC multicentre study in India and Africa. Int J Cancer 2004; 110:907–913.
29. Sarian LO, Derchain SF, Naud P, et al. Evaluation of visual inspection with acetic acid (VIA), Lugol's iodine (VILI), cervical cytology and HPV testing as cervical screening tools in Latin America. This report refers to partial results from the LAMS (Latin AMerican Screening) study. J Med Screen 2005; 12:142–149.
30. Sankaranarayanan R, Nene BM, Shastri SS et al. HPV screening for cervical cancer in rural India. N Engl J Med 2009; 360:1385–1394.
31. Sankaranarayanan R, Rajkumar R, Esmy PO, et al. Effectiveness, safety and acceptability of 'see and treat' with cryotherapy by nurses in a cervical screening study in India. Br J Cancer 2007; 96:738–743.
32. Sankaranarayanan R, Nene BM, Dinshaw KA, et al. A cluster randomized controlled trial of visual, cytology and human papillomavirus screening for cancer of the cervix in rural India. Int J Cancer 2005; 116:617–623.
33. Denny L, Kuhn L, De Souza M, et al. Screen-and-treat approaches for cervical cancer prevention in low-resource settings: a randomized controlled trial. JAMA 2005; 294:2173–2181.
34. Kitchener HC, Denton K, Soldan K, et al. Developing role of HPV in cervical cancer prevention. BMJ 2013; 347:f4781.
35. Finan RR, Irani-Hakime N, Tamim H, et al. Molecular diagnosis of human papillomavirus: comparison between cervical and vaginal sampling. Infect Dis Obstet Gynecol 2001; 9:119–122.
36. Wright TC Jr, Denny L, Kuhn L, et al. HPV DNA testing of self-collected vaginal samples compared with cytologic screening to detect cervical cancer. JAMA 2000; 283:81–86.
37. Sellors JW, Lorincz AT, Mahony JB, et al. Comparison of self-collected vaginal, vulvar and urine samples with physician-collected cervical samples for human papillomavirus testing to detect high-grade squamous intraepithelial lesions. CMAJ 2000; 163:513–518.
38. Stenvall H, Wikstrom I, Wilander E. Human papilloma virus testing of vaginal smear obtained with a novel self-sampling device. Acta Derm Venereol 2006; 86:465–467.
39. Stenkvist B, Soderstrom J. Reasons for cervical cancer despite extensive screening. J Med Screen 1996; 3:204–207.
40. Agreda PM, Beitman GH, Gutierrez EC, et al. Long-term stability of human genomic and human papillomavirus DNA stored in BD SurePath and Hologic PreservCyt liquid-based cytology media. J Clin Microbiol 2013; 51:2702–2706.
41. Petignat P, Faltin DL, Bruchim I, et al. Are self-collected samples comparable to physician-collected cervical specimens for human papillomavirus DNA testing? A systematic review and meta-analysis. Gynecol Oncol 2007; 105:530–535.

42. Cattani P, Siddu A, D'Onghia S, et al. RNA (E6 and E7) assays versus DNA (E6 and E7) assays for risk evaluation for women infected with human papillomavirus. J Clin Microbiol 2009; 47:2136–2141.
43. Rijkaart DC, Heideman DA, Coupe VM, et al. High-risk human papillomavirus (hrHPV) E6/E7 mRNA testing by PreTect HPV-Proofer for detection of cervical high-grade intraepithelial neoplasia and cancer among hrHPV DNA-positive women with normal cytology. J Clin Microbiol 2012; 50:2390–2396.
44. Benevolo M, Vocaturo A, Caraceni D, et al. Sensitivity, specificity, and clinical value of human papillomavirus (HPV) E6/E7 mRNA assay as a triage test for cervical cytology and HPV DNA test. J Clin Microbiol 2011; 49:2643–2650.
45. Wang SM, Colombara D, Shi JF, et al. Six-year regression and progression of cervical lesions of different human papillomavirus viral loads in varied histological diagnoses. Int J Gynecol Cancer 2013; 23:716–723.
46. Gustinucci D, Passamonti B, Cesarini E, et al. Role of p16(INK4a) cytology testing as an adjunct to enhance the diagnostic specificity and accuracy in human papillomavirus-positive women within an organized cervical cancer screening program. Acta Cytol 2012; 56:506–514.
47. Roelens J, Reuschenbach M, von Knebel Doeberitz M, et al. p16INK4a immunocytochemistry versus human papillomavirus testing for triage of women with minor cytologic abnormalities: a systematic review and meta-analysis. Cancer Cytopathol 2012; 120:294–307.
48. Petry KU, Schmidt D, Scherbring S, et al. Triaging Pap cytology negative, HPV positive cervical cancer screening results with p16/Ki-67 Dual-stained cytology. Gynecol Oncol 2011; 121:505–509.

Chapter 11

Domestic violence and its relevance in obstetrics and gynaecology

Tonye Wokoma, Stephen Lindow

INTRODUCTION

There is a growing and diverse body of research on domestic violence that covers a broad range of issues including global incidences [1,2], social indicators and risk factors associated with domestic violence [3–5]. Strategies for identification and support as well as implications in obstetrics and gynaecology have become increasingly important. This chapter examines domestic violence and its relevance to obstetrics and gynaecology.

Definition of domestic violence

Domestic violence is defined as 'any incident or pattern of incidents of controlling, coercive, threatening behaviour, violence or abuse between those aged 16 or over who are, or have been, intimate partners or family members regardless of gender or sexuality. The abuse can encompass, but is not limited to, psychological, physical, sexual, financial and emotional abuse' according to the United Kingdom Home Office, 2013.

PREVALENCE

Domestic violence is a significant global health issue [6]. It is estimated that over 35% of the worldwide female population have experienced some form of violence from their intimate partners and/or significant others [2]. Though domestic violence is a widespread public health concern, there are significant variations in the estimated prevalence not just internationally but also within national boundaries [7]. For example, in the United States of America (USA), the incidence rates of lifetime domestic violence are reported to be 1.9% in Washington but up to 70% within the Hispanic Latinas community in South Eastern USA [7]. Evidence from developing countries suggests that anywhere from 10% to 60% of married women of reproductive age report having ever experienced some form of domestic violence [8]. Domestic violence by a current or former partner is the most common cause of injury to women, comprising 21% of traumatic injuries [9]. A Nordic questionnaire study

Tonye Wokoma MBBS MRCOG MFSRH, Conifer House, Wilberforce Centre, Hull, UK . Email: tonye.wokoma@nhs.net (for correspondence)

Stephen Lindow MB Chb MMed MD FRCOG FCOG(SA) FRCPI, Sidra Medical and Research Center, Doha, Qatar

exploring abusive experiences showed that 20% of female respondents over the age of 18 years attending gynaecology clinics reported having endured death threats during their lifetime [10]. Domestic violence may be lethal with murder a potential consequence [10,11].

Despite the imprecision about quantifying the scale of the problem, it is clear that domestic violence is a significant, pervasive societal problem and has implications in general health care. In obstetric and gynaecological practice, domestic violence is particularly relevant with the highest average lifetime incidence of a broad range of domestic violence being reported in obstetrics, gynaecology and psychiatric clinics [11]. However, it is possible that the incidence of domestic violence in female populations sampled from outpatient clinics may overestimate the general female incidence because women with a history of domestic violence may be more likely to consult their doctors [13] and present with gynaecological problems [14]. Despite this caveat, the prevalence and severity of emotional, physical, and sexual abuse are high in women attending gynaecology clinics [10].

Professionals involved in antenatal care need to be vigilant to domestic violence. Abuse in a relationship usually precedes a pregnancy but for a significant number of women the abuse may start for the first time in pregnancy [15,16] although for a minority of women, there may be a reduction in domestic violence during pregnancy [17,18].

IMPACT ON HEALTH

The impact of domestic violence on women's health is wide ranging and is often associated with adverse long-term effects on general, reproductive and mental health [17,18]. Deleterious effects on well-being may continue even after the violence has ended [19] with ongoing poor health status, reduced quality of life and increased use of health care services [13]. Injuries arising from physical violence are the most obvious consequence of domestic violence; however, intimate partner abuse is associated with much more complex physical health impacts [19].

Gynaecology

It is important to recognise that domestic violence is a multifactorial problem and is linked to gynaecological morbidity. There appears to be a lack of identification of most victims of domestic violence by their gynaecologists [10]. A study from the United Kingdom (UK) found that women with a history of domestic violence were more likely to complain of lower abdominal pain, dyspareunia, dysmenorrhoea and bowel symptoms [14] They were also more likely to have smear abnormalities and worry about cancer [14]. High incidence rates of domestic violence have also been reported among women who attend clinics for severe premenstrual syndrome [20].

It has been proposed that plausible mechanisms through which domestic violence may influence gynaecologic morbidity include physical trauma, psychological stress or transmission of sexually transmitted infections [8]. Several studies show that pregnant women who had experienced partner's physical or sexual violence or both were significantly more likely to report having had at least one induced abortion than women who had never experienced domestic violence. Women's ability to control their fertility may be restricted when subjected to a climate of fear and control within abusive relationships [21]. Lack of fertility control can lead to unintended pregnancies, which are also associated with adverse outcomes for both women and their infant's health, especially in developing countries [21].

Obstetrics

A recent UK study compared self-reported rates of domestic violence between pregnant women in the first trimester attending for antenatal care with women attending termination of pregnancy clinics. Those women requesting termination of pregnancy were five to six times more likely to have suffered emotional and physical abuse than women attending antenatal clinics [22]. However, this study did not implicate domestic violence to be a factor in the choice for pregnancy termination [22].

Domestic violence in pregnant women is thought to be as prevalent as other more commonly screened for complications such as gestational diabetes and pre-eclampsia [3]. According to the confidential enquiry into maternal deaths in the UK during 2006–2008, 34 women who died from any cause had features of domestic violence and in the 11 cases of murder all but two women were murdered by a partner or family member [23]. In addition to the direct physical and mental health consequences for women suffering domestic violence, it is important to appreciate that the incidence of adverse pregnancy outcomes has increased in victims of such abuse [24,25].

Several studies show an increased incidence for both maternal and fetal adverse health outcomes [25,26] including increased incidence of preterm labour or delivery, operative vaginal or caesarean delivery, puerperal pyrexia, breastfeeding problems, anxiety and depression. The fetus may suffer from maladaptive growth and development [27], and poor neonatal outcomes include low birthweight, higher rates of birth asphyxia and neonatal death [25]. The impact of domestic violence on pregnancy outcome is complicated by its co-occurrence with depression and alcohol use. A significant association has been demonstrated between domestic violence and illicit drug use (16.7%) and active smoking (22%), both behaviours being established risk factors for preterm birth and low birthweight [28]. Furthermore, domestic and sexual abuse may lead to sexually transmitted diseases in pregnancy including human immunodeficiency virus (HIV) with the potential for vertical transmission to the baby [29].

Domestic violence is also known to have a negative impact on the mental health of women [30] with several investigations showing that female victims of violence by their partners are at risk of developing psychological problems including depression in pregnancy, postpartum depression and post-traumatic stress disorders [30]. The psychological effects of domestic abuse on women are substantial and varied. They include fear, an increased susceptibility to misusing drugs, alcohol or prescribed antidepressants, depression/poor mental health, wanting to commit or actually committing suicide, sleep disturbances, post-traumatic stress disorder, anger, guilt, loss of self-confidence, feelings of dependency, loss of hope, feelings of isolation, low self-worth, panic or anxiety, eating disorders [31].

SOCIAL INDICATORS AND RISK FACTORS FOR DOMESTIC VIOLENCE

Domestic violence occurs across the whole society regardless of age, ethnicity, religion, social class and income or where people live [31]. Markers for domestic violence are imprecise; however, there may be an increased risk for some particularly vulnerable groups such as women who are transient, women in low socioeconomic groups and women with mental health problems. Domestic violence in English-speaking countries may also be difficult to identify in women where English is not a first language [23,31]. Other risk factors included for domestic violence in pregnancy include serious levels of violence preconception, feelings of inadequacy, jealousy and controlling behaviour, partner intravenous drug abuse.

Women who are victims of domestic violence hardly share their experiences without structured and purposeful prompting [32], and therefore there is the risk of failing to identify domestic violence and the formulation of misdiagnoses from the presenting complaints [10]. However, women find it acceptable to be routinely asked about domestic violence [33]. Health professionals caring for pregnant women should remain alert to the possibility of domestic violence especially in women with health conditions, behaviours and relationships that may indicate possible domestic violence.

Factors that may alert the clinician to domestic violence in a pregnant woman:
- Late booker/poor attender
- Repeat attendances for minor injuries
- Unexplained admissions
- Depression/anxiety/self-harm
- Injuries of different ages with minimisation
- Sexually transmitted infections/urinary tract infections/vaginal infections
- Poor obstetric history
- Domineering partner

The main barriers to screening include lack of training, lack of time and a lack of knowledge about appropriate interventions if domestic violence is revealed. Fear of offending the patient or her partner is often also mentioned by health care professionals as a barrier to screening for domestic violence [34].

Health care professionals who see women with domestic violence should focus in the first instance on the woman's immediate safety and that of her children, if she has any. She needs to be given appropriate information and referred to relevant agencies that provide support for women, such as shelters and refuges, and domestic violence helplines. Support and reassurance are vital and health care professional must remain nonjudgemental [31].

Evidence supporting the effectiveness of routine screening of asymptomatic women in improving health status is lacking. However, identification of domestic violence within specific contexts and provision of targeted interventions may provide health benefits [35]. Antenatal care is one such situation where the screening for domestic violence and provision of substantive tailored interventions may have a favourable impact on recurrence of domestic violence and maternal and infant outcomes [28,36].

A randomised controlled trial (RCT) was performed in 1044 pregnant African-American women who were assigned either an integrated cognitive behavioural intervention or normal care. The intervention was performed at routine antenatal appointments by Masters-level social workers or psychologists and involved specific, evidence-based, interventions for the designated psychobehavioural risks [28]. There was a significant reduction in the rates of intimate partner violence; the odds of further episodes of minor or severe physical violence within the antenatal or postnatal period were halved. Furthermore, improvements in obstetric outcomes were also seen. These included a significant reduction in very low birthweight (<1.5 kg) and very preterm delivery (<33 weeks) and an increase in gestational age at delivery (38.2 vs. 36.9 weeks) between the experimental group receiving cognitive behavioural therapy and the control group receiving standard care. Thus, screening for domestic violence in pregnancy as well as for psychological (e.g. depression) and behavioural risks (e.g. smoking, alcohol abuse, illicit drug use) and providing targeted similar cognitive behavioural intervention appears to provide benefits on rates of recurrent violence and pregnancy outcomes. More than half the women suffering domestic violence in this study reported depression. The authors concluded that by addressing domestic violence and depression together may have helped women implement strategies suggested to them to assess risks, consider preventive options and develop safety plans [28].

Another RCT set in Hong Kong also lends support to the notion that specific psychobehavioural interventions in pregnancy may help improve maternal outcomes. In this RCT, 110 pregnant women with a history of abuse by their intimate partners were randomised between empowerment training specially designed for Chinese abused pregnant women or standard care for abused women. The trial showed that women receiving empowerment training had significantly higher physical functioning and improved role limitation scores due to physical and emotional problems as measured by the SF 36 quality of life instrument. Obstetric outcomes were not reported but there was less postnatal depression recorded in the experimental group. Minor abuse was significantly reduced, although there was no reduction in severe abuse [36].

This evidence to support a strategy of screening and treatment within pregnancy mandates obstetricians, midwives, health service managers and others involved with caring for pregnant women to implement effective management strategies for domestic violence. These plans should involve seeing women on their own at some clinic visits with sensitive routine enquiry about domestic violence and appropriate referral for psychobehavioural intervention. Referral pathways need to be agreed and staff need to be educated and equipped to deal with this issue.

CONCLUSION

Domestic violence is a serious public health issue and there is still a long way to go with reducing the incidence of abuse and adverse health impacts upon sufferers. Strategies for identification and support are well described. There is a need for all agencies to work together in a holistic way to best manage the short- and long-term health impact of domestic violence on women and children. Current research indicates that pregnancy may be a unique time in a woman's medical life when the attending medical staff can address the problem of domestic violence. Therefore, screening and treatment may be uniquely applied to this group of consultations. The health benefits may not only include a reduction in the frequency and severity of domestic violence but also improvements in obstetric and neonatal outcomes. Further research into prevention of domestic violence is required as well as the development of effective interventions to improve general health for victims of abuse and to reduce associated obstetric and gynaecological morbidity where encountered.

Key points for clinical practice

- Screening and interventions for domestic violence in the antenatal period is effective in reducing the recurrence of domestic violence.
- Women with associated depression and substance misuse issues should be referred along agreed pathways for psycho-behavioural intervention. This improves obstetric and neonatal outcomes.
- Regular staff training and update to enhance staff confidence in identifying and managing domestic violence.

REFERENCES

1.   Singh BP, Singh KK, Singh N. Couple interaction and predicting vulnerability to domestic violence J Interpers Violence 2014; 29: 2304.
2.   World Health Organization (WHO), Department of Reproductive Health and Research, London School of Hygiene and Tropical Medicine, South African Medical Research Council. Global and regional estimates of violence against women. Prevalence and health effects of intimate partner violence and non-partner sexual violence. Geneva; WHO, 2013.
3.   Chatha SA, Ahmad K, Sheikh KS. Socio-economic status and domestic violence: a study on married women in urban Lahore, Pakistan. South Asian Studies 2014; 29:229-237.
4.   Pestka K and Wendt S Belonging: women living with intellectual disabilities and experiences of domestic violence. Disabil Soc 2014; 29: 1031–1045.
5.   Mishra A, Patne S, Tiwari R, et al A cross-sectional study to find out the prevalence of different types of domestic violence in Gwalior city and to identify the various risk and protective factors for domestic violence. Indian J Community Med 2014; 39:21–25.
6.   McGarry J, Westbury M, Kench S, et al Responding to domestic violence in acute hospital settings. Nurs Stand 2014; 28:47–50.
7.   Alhabib S, Nur U, Jones R. Domestic violence against women: systematic review of prevalence studies. J Fam Violence 2010; 25:369–382.
8.   Stephenson R, Koenig MA, Ahmed S. Domestic violence and symptoms of gynecologic morbidity among women in North India. International family planning perspectives, 2006; 32:201–208.
9.   Guth AA, and Pachter HL. Domestic violence and the trauma surgeon. Am J Surg 2000; 179:134-140.
10. Wijma B, Schei B, Swahnberg K, et al Emotional, physical, and sexual abuse in patients visiting gynecology clinics: a Nordic cross-sectional study. Lancet 2003; 361:2107–2113.
11. Crawford M, Gartner R, Dawson M. Intimate femicide in Ontario, 1974–1994. Toronto; Women We Honour Action Committee, 1997.
12. Oram S, Trevillion K, Feder G, et al Prevalence of experiences of domestic violence among psychiatric patients: systematic review. Br J Psychiatry 2013; 202:94–99.
13. Campbell JC. Health consequences of intimate partner violence. Lancet 2002; 359:1331.
14. John RR, Johnson JK, Kukreja SS, et al Domestic violence: prevalence and association with gynaecological symptoms. BJOG 2004; 111:1128–1132.
15. Johnson JK, Haider F, Ellis K, et al. The prevalence of domestic violence in pregnant women. BJOG 2003; 110:272-275.
16. Lewis G and Drife J. Why mothers die 2000-2002, the sixth report. London; Royal College of Obstetricians and Gynaecologists, 2004.
17. Goodman P. Intimate Partner Violence and Pregnancy. In C. Mitchell and D. Anglin: Intimate Partner Violence, A Health Based Perspective. New York; Oxford University Press, 2009.
18. Garcia-Moreno C, Jansen H, Ellsberg M, et al. WHO multi-country study on women's health and domestic violence against women: summary report of initial results on prevalence, health outcomes and women's responses. Geneva; World Health Organization, 2005.
19. Fraser K. Domestic violence and women's physical health. Sydney; Australian Domestic and Family Violence Clearinghouse, 2003
20. Golding JM, Taylor DL, Menard L, et al Prevalence of sexual abuse history in a sample of women seeking treatment for premenstrual syndrome. J Psychosom Obstet Gynaecol 2000; 21:69–80.
21. Pallitto CC, Campbell JC, O'Campo P. Is intimate partner violence associated with unintended pregnancy? A review of the literature. Trauma Violence Abuse 2005; 6:217–235.
22. Wokoma T, Jampala M, Bexhell H, et al A comparative study of the prevalence of domestic violence in women requesting a termination of pregnancy and those attending the antenatal clinic. BJOG 2014; 121:627–633.
23. Saving Mothers' Lives. Reviewing maternal deaths to make motherhood safer: 2006–2008 The Eighth Report of the Confidential Enquiries into Maternal Deaths in the United Kingdom. BJOG 2011; 118:148.
24. Yost NP, Bloom SL, McIntire DD, et al A prospective observational study of domestic violence during pregnancy. Obstet Gynecol 2005; 106:61–65.
25. Enang EE, Adegboyega AF, Abiodun PA, et al Domestic violence and obstetric outcome among pregnant women in Ilorin, North Central Nigeria. Int J Gynaecol Obstet 2014; 125:170–171.
26. Parsons LH, Harper MA. Violent maternal deaths in North Carolina. Obstet Gynecol 1999; 94:990–993.

27. Kim H, Mandell M, Crandall C, et al Antenatal psychiatric illness and adequacy of prenatal care in an ethnical diverse inner-city obstetric population. Arch Womens Ment Health 2006; 9:103–107.
28. Kiely M, El-Mohandes A, El-Khorazaty M, et al An integrated intervention to reduce intimate partner violence in pregnancy: a randomized controlled trial. Obstet Gynecol 2010; 115:273–283.
29. Maman S, Campbell JC, Sweat M, et al The intersection of HIV and violence: directions for future research and interventions. Soc Sci Med 2000; 50:459–478.
30. Almeida CP, Cunha FF, Pires EP, et al Common mental disorders in pregnancy in the context of interpartner violence. J Psychiatr Ment Health Nurs 2013; 20: 419–425.
31. Department of Health. Responding to Domestic Violence. a handbook for health professionals. London, Department of Health, 2005.
32. D'Avolio D, Hawkins JW, Haggerty LA, et al Screening for abuse: barriers and opportunities. Health Care Women Int 2001; 22:349–362.
33. Howe A, Crilly M, Fairhurst R. Acceptability of asking patients about violence in accident and emergency. Emerg Med J 2002; 19:138–140.
34. Elliot L, Nerney M, Jones T, et al Barriers to screening for domestic violence. J Gen Intern med 2002; 17:112–116.
35. Jewkes R. Intimate partner violence: the end of routine screening. Lancet 2013; 382:190–191.
36. Tiwari A, Leung WC, Leung TW, et al A randomised controlled trial of empowerment training for Chinese abused pregnant women in Hong Kong. BJOG 2005; 112:1249–1256.

Chapter 12

Pregnancy after assisted reproductive technology

Jinny Yuting Foo, William Ledger, Michael Chapman

INTRODUCTION

The use of assisted reproductive technology (ART) is increasing worldwide. Births are now estimated to be in excess of five million. In Australia, almost 4% of all births are a result of ART [1] with the average age of women undertaking ART cycles with their own oocytes being 36 years [2]. This review will summarise the potential risks that a woman who successfully undertakes fertility treatment with ART may face in the course of her pregnancy, as compared to their counterparts who conceive naturally.

STILLBIRTH AND NEONATAL DEATH

A retrospective Australian study of pregnancies in women conceiving after ART has shown that they are nearly twice as likely to result in a stillbirth compared with those pregnancies conceived naturally [3]. This increase in risk also applied to women who conceived naturally but had a history of infertility. Furthermore, live born singletons were more likely to die within the neonatal period if they were conceived through ART as compared to those who were conceived spontaneously [3]. The worldwide epidemic of multiple pregnancies arising from ART, with some countries recording twinning rates in excess of 40%, exaggerates the perinatal risks even further.

In contrast to fresh embryo transfer cycles with in-vitro fertilisation (IVF) or intra-cytoplasmic insemination (ICSI), frozen transfer cycles did not seem to be associated with an increased risk of stillbirths [3]. The reasons why frozen embryo transfer appears to result in better outcomes are not known. It has been suggested that the self-selection effect of freezing filters out developmentally compromised embryos that are less likely to survive [3]. Another theory is the iatrogenic asynchrony seen in a fresh embryo transfer between embryonic development and endometrial receptivity that may affect implantation [4]. This

Jinny Yuting Foo BMed MRMed, Women's and Children's Health, St George Hospital, Sydney, Australia

William Ledger MA DPhil(Oxon) MB ChB FRCOG FRANZCOG CREI, School of Women's and Children's Health, University of New South Wales, Sydney, Australia

Michael Chapman MBBS FRCOG FRANZCOG MD CREI, School of Women's and Children's Health, University of New South Wales, Sydney, Australia. Email: M.Chapman@unsw.edu.au (for correspondence)

is possibly due to the endometrial receptivity from excessive estrogen and progesterone due to ovarian stimulation in a fresh embryo transfer; whereas a frozen cycle with a more natural uterine environment may be more favourable for development [4].

PERINATAL MORBIDITY

In addition to perinatal mortality, perinatal morbidity is also increased in women undergoing ART. They are more likely to have very low birthweight infants or small-for-gestational age (SGA) babies even in singleton pregnancies with an estimated 13% of babies born after ART having a birthweight of <2500 g [2]. The risk of very preterm birth (<32 weeks' gestation) or preterm birth (<37 weeks' gestation) following ART is increased two- to threefold [5], a complication with known implications to future child development [6]. The exact mechanism that causes prematurity and low birthweight in singleton pregnancies following ART is unclear. It is interesting to note that the risks of preterm birth and low birthweight appear to be more significant with female-factor infertility [6,7]. Moreover, the risk of preterm birth and low birthweight also applies to women with a previously recorded infertility diagnosis, who conceive naturally [3]; a risk that seems to be accentuated in women requiring oocyte donation [8].

IVF with frozen cycles does not have an increased risk of neonatal death, very preterm births or infants with very low birthweight. Yet, the risk of SGA, preterm births and low birth weight remains [3]. ICSI with frozen embryo transfer does not seem to have an association with any adverse perinatal outcomes. Indeed, these infants may prove to be heavier and more likely to result in large-for-gestational age babies as compared with fertile naturally conceived contemporaries [3]. Overall, no difference in the mean gestational age at birth between babies resulting from frozen or fresh oocytes has been reported [9].

Women with twin pregnancies either as a result from ART or spontaneous conception following an infertility diagnosis also showed a similar trend towards very preterm births, infants with very low birthweight and neonatal deaths [3].

EARLY PREGNANCY COMPLICATIONS

Pregnancies after ART are believed to have a 20–34% increased risk of spontaneous miscarriage compared to spontaneous conceptions. Furthermore, there appears to be a positive correlation between the risk of spontaneous abortions and the intensity of ovarian stimulation [10]. A recent study, albeit with small number of patients, has shown no difference in the miscarriage rates when comparing couples who have had both fresh and frozen cycles [9]. A recent prospective cohort study comparing spontaneous and ART pregnancies found no increase in miscarriage but did note an increased risk of vaginal bleeding during pregnancy in women who conceive after ART. This was mostly seen in the first trimester and appeared to be accentuated in the presence of a diagnosis of polycystic ovarian syndrome (PCOS) [13].

When evaluating these data, there are certain caveats to be considered. These include the fact that women who undergo ART are on average 5 years older than those who conceive naturally [1], which could be a confounding factor for any apparent increase in miscarriage risk. It should also be appreciated that women with subfertility issues who spontaneously conceive appear to have a similar risk of miscarriage compared to those who undertake ART [10]. These observations suggest that the underlying fertility status rather than the ART may be the important aetiological factor.

Aneuploidy is likely to result in implantation failure or miscarriage with a quoted 40% likelihood of chromosomal abnormality with two IVF failures and rising to 50% with five IVF failures [11]. The observed trend towards increased early pregnancy loss may be reversed in time with advances in pre-implantation genetic diagnosis that can be offered to select chromosomally normal embryos and to improve embryo selection thereby increasing subsequent pregnancy rates. It has also recently documented that array-comparative genomic hybridisation used together with morphology screening for the selection of blastocysts during ART results in higher clinical pregnancy rates, as compared to morphology screening alone [12]. Such screening reduces genetic abnormalities in the offspring.

PLACENTATION ISSUES

There is a higher rate of placenta praevia and placental abruption in ART pregnancies when compared with the non-IVF pregnancies [14,15]. Two theories have been postulated concerning the cause of placenta praevia after ART: (i) metabolic changes in an embryo during culture or (ii) uterine stimulation causing contractility during embryo transfer leading to increased frequency of implantation in the lower segment [15]. Further research into this area is needed. When comparing frozen and fresh cycles of ART, frozen cycles are associated with a decreased risk of antepartum haemorrhage after 20 weeks' gestation, with an absolute 2% decrease in risk. In particular, a thawed frozen embryo transfer is reported to lower the risk of placenta praevia and abruption [4]. A recent study suggests reduced endometrial thickness during ART to be associated with a higher incidence of placenta praevia [30].

MEDICAL DISORDERS OF PREGNANCY

A prospective cohort study published in 2013 showed a trend towards an increased risk of hypertensive disorders in pregnancy with ART [13]. This risk was increased by 55% [10] following ART and was particularly high after oocyte donation [8], which may be related to altered immunological processes associated with the two 'foreign' genotypes to which the mother is exposed [16]. The impact of frozen versus fresh ART on pregnancy-induced hypertension remains unresolved. Besides the different assisted techniques used for conception, factors underlying subfertility may also affect the likelihood of developing hypertensive disorders in pregnancy [10].

There may also be a trend towards an increased risk of gestational diabetes in both singleton and twin pregnancies after ART but this contention remains controversial [17]. In part, this may relate to the background risk inherent in the infertile sub population with insulin resistance and PCOS.

Any increased risk of developing medical disorders in pregnancy associated with ART may be attributed in part to the women's age. Women who resort to ART are more likely to be older. In Australia, the average age of women giving birth after ART is 5 years greater than for naturally conceiving mothers [1]. The previously discussed predisposition to preterm delivery in ART pregnancies may relate to occult or manifest medical disorders such as hypertension, heart disease and insulin resistance [18].

SINGLE VERSUS DOUBLE EMBRYO TRANSFER

Regardless of the method of conception, it is well known that twins and higher order pregnancies result in more maternal and neonatal complications than singleton pregnancies. Complications include an increased risk of pre-eclampsia, postpartum haemorrhage, preterm birth, perinatal mortality and perinatal morbidity of survivors [17]. Multiple birth rates are higher following double embryo transfer compared to single embryo transfers; and twins have worse perinatal outcomes compared to singletons. In addition, live born singletons resulting from a double embryo transfer are also at increased risk of poor perinatal outcome; they are 15% more likely to have lower birthweight neonates and 13% more likely to have a preterm birth when compared to singletons conceived by single embryo transfers [19].

The fetal mortality rate for singletons conceived following a double embryo transfer has been estimated to be 10.9 per 1000 compared to 8.9 per 1000 for singletons conceived following a single embryo transfer. However, the observed increase in fetal mortality did not reach statistical significance. Live birth rates in fresh and frozen single embryo transfer are comparable to double embryo transfer [17].

CAESAREAN SECTION

The caesarean section delivery rate following ART is 49.5% in Australia [2]. In other regional Assisted Reproduction Databases, such as in North America and the United Kingdom, statistics on the method of birth are not available [20]. A Swedish register has reported that the likelihood of caesarean section was increased by 40% for singletons and 20% for multiple births [20]. The higher rate of caesarean section deliveries following ART may result from maternal anxiety and patient preference rather than from clear obstetric indications. A meta-analysis has reported a slight increase in frequency of both elective and emergency caesarean sections following oocyte donation [8] and in frozen ART cycles as compared with fresh ART cycles [4]. The average maternal age at delivery for women receiving ART is 5 years older than the average maternal age at delivery in Australia. This is another possible explanation for the rise in caesarean section rates in women receiving ART [2]. Also contributing to the increased caesarean section rate is the higher rate of multiple births following ART. This contribution is small in Australia where multiple pregnancy rates are only 6.9% due to a 72% single embryo transfer rate. However, the influence of multiple pregnancy on caesarean section rates is greater in the United Kingdom and United States of America where twinning rates following ART are higher following ART at 20% and >30% respectively [17].

CONGENITAL MALFORMATIONS

A number of studies and two large meta-analyses have demonstrated an increased risk of congenital malformation in children following IVF and ICSI compared with children who are naturally conceived. These include neural tube defects, cardiovascular defects, gastrointestinal defects, genitourinary defects and musculoskeletal defects [7,17,21]. However, expanding the scope of birth defects to include cerebral palsy up until the age of 5, an Australian birth registry has demonstrated that there was no difference in the rates of birth defects following IVF after adjusting for potential confounding factors such as maternal age, patient demographics and maternal conditions in pregnancy. However, ICSI had a statistically higher adjusted odds ratio (aOR) for birth defects [aOR 1.57; 95% confidence interval (CI) 1.30–1.90] [22]. However, the increased risk of ICSI was not observed in women becoming pregnant after transfer of cryopreserved embryos [21]. The overall prevalence of congenital malformations also appears to increase with increasing time to achieve a pregnancy whether conceived naturally or with ART [9,22,23,24].

No difference in birth defects up until 5 years of age was observed in the same Australian study between twins conceived from ART versus twins conceived naturally [22]. This is likely due to the fact that twins conceived via ART are more likely to be dizygotic than those conceived naturally because it is mainly the monozygotic twins that are at increased risk of birth defects [22].

GROWTH AND DEVELOPMENT OF CHILDREN

With respect to the growth and development of children born from ART, recent studies and systematic reviews have negated any concerns in the neurodevelopmental status of these children. Children born after ART appear to have a normal progress in their motor and cognitive ability as compared to their counterparts who were conceived naturally [21]. Studies on psychomotor development have shown no deficits, but analysis of cognitive and behavioural development is lacking in infants and teenagers [25]. Nevertheless, most of these studies are based on toddlers and children in their middle childhood and as such, more complex cognitive function may not yet be displayed. Although studies have not documented an increased risk for intellectual disability, there was an increased risk of suspected developmental delay in children whose mothers were younger than 30 years old [26]. It has been suggested that parents who have undergone IVF may be more anxious about their child's well-being than parents who have conceived naturally [26]. Similarly, parents who have conceived through IVF may seek medical help more readily than others for less subtle signs of mild attention deficit hyperactivity disorder (ADHD) or Asperger syndrome [26].

To date, ART has not specifically been associated with an increased autism, sensory impairment and intellectual disability [26,27]. However, there is a small association between ovulation induction with a small increased incidence of a mental disorder, autism spectrum disorder or Asperger syndrome, ADHD, conduct, emotional or social disorder [28].

The risk of cerebral palsy appears to be affected by other confounders such as multiple births and their inherent risk of preterm birth [26]. This is largely associated with parental subfertility [26]. However, with the reduction of double embryo transfers and the associated morbidity of multiple births, the rates of cerebral palsy may start to fall [26].

No difference in postnatal growth, pubertal development and bone mineralisation between children who were naturally conceived and those conceived after IVF has been observed [21,28].

CHILDHOOD MEDICAL PROBLEMS

Although earlier studies have suggested that there is no increased need to access health care facilities for children conceived from ART in the neonatal period, recent studies have shown that children born after ART have more admissions to hospital than children conceived naturally up until school age [26]. No difference is seen from 7 to 11 years of age [26].

There is some evidence to suggest a difference in the cardio-metabolic status of children born after IVF such as higher arterial blood pressures, elevated fasting blood glucose levels and a tendency towards an increased total body fat content. This is hypothesised to be because of a vascular dysfunction following hormonal stimulation during ART [29]. There is uncertainty regarding the current implications of these isolated findings with further research required. Regardless, there is still concern of the associated long-term consequences of the observed cardio-metabolic changes following ART [21,27].

The prevalence of childhood asthma and bronchitis is greater in children born after ART as compared to children who were conceived naturally [26]. This association was also seen in mothers with fecundity problems and previous miscarriages [26]. Children born after ART appeared to be at a greater risk of epilepsy than children who were conceived naturally [26]. However, this difference was not statistically significant once adjustments for confounding factors were made [26]. The risk of childhood cancer in children born after ART is uncertain and requires further research.

CONCLUSION

The majority of research into perinatal and pregnancy outcomes after ART has been based on observational studies and retrospective data collection, with risks of bias and confounding. Although there are reassuring data on the growth and neurodevelopmental status of children and safety data on effects of cryopreservation, it is essential to regard any ART pregnancy as high risk with increased risks of miscarriage, placentation problems, maternal medical disorders, caesarean section, prematurity, low birthweight, perinatal morbidity and mortality. Risks associated with pregnancy are further increased after oocyte donation, with its inherent risk of hypertensive disorders, antepartum haemorrhage and increased perinatal morbidity.

In addition to the pregnancy risks that are associated with successful ART, it appears that women with a personal history of subfertility who conceive naturally are also faced with the similar problems [22]. Thus, it may well be that any increased risks in pregnancy may not be related to the ART intervention per se. That said, it remains necessary to counsel couples concerning the risks of ART, particularly before multiple embryo transfer, but also to educate them on the perinatal and obstetric implications of ART and subfertility. Ongoing research is needed to help us to provide optimal fertility treatment and management in the future.

Key points for clinical practice

- ART pregnancy is a high-risk pregnancy.
- Women undergoing ART are more likely to experience a stillbirth or neonatal death as compared to women who conceive naturally.
- Women who conceived by ART are more likely to have a low birthweight or very low birthweight baby.
- The risk of preterm delivery before 32 weeks and 37 weeks is increased by two- to threefold in women seeking ART treatment.

- Early pregnancy problems such as miscarriages and vaginal bleeding in the first trimester are more common in women undergoing ART.

- Higher rates of placenta praevia and abruption are observed in IVF pregnancies compared to non-IVF pregnancies.

- Increased medical complications in pregnancy are noted in women who conceived through IVF. These include hypertensive disorders in pregnancy and gestational diabetes and may be age-related.

- Women with a history of subfertility who conceive naturally appear to have similar overall risks associated with pregnancy compared to women undergoing ART.

- Caesarean section rates in women who have had an IVF pregnancy are higher than those who have naturally conceived.

- The neonatal outcomes following ART pregnancies are reassuring compared to the spontaneously conceived population, but long-term follow-up studies of these children into adulthood are required.

REFERENCES

1. Li Z, Zeki R, Hilder L, et al. 2013. Australia's mothers and babies 2011. Perinatal statistics series no. 28. Cat no. PER 39. Canberra: AIHW National Perinatal Epidemiology and Statistics Unit.
2. Macaldowie A, Wang YA, Chambers GM, et al. 2013. Assisted reproductive technology in Australia and New Zealand 2011. Sydney: National Perinatal Epidemiology and Statistics Unit, the University of New South Wales.
3. Marino JL, Moore VM, Willson KJ, et al. Perinatal outcomes by mode of assisted conception and sub-fertility in an Australian data linkage cohort. PLOS ONE 2014; 9:e80398.
4. Maheshwari A, Pandey S, Shetty A, et al. Obstetric and perinatal outcomes in singleton pregnancies resulting from the transfer of frozen thawed versus fresh embryos generated through in vitro fertilization treatment: a systematic review and meta-analysis. Fertil Steril 2014; 98:368–377.
5. Helmerhorst FM, Perquin DAM, Donker D, et al. Perinatal outcome of singletons and twins after assisted conception: a systematic review of controlled studies. BMJ 2004; 328:261–264.
6. Ceelen M, van Weissenbruch MM, Vermeiden JPW, et al. Growth and development of children born after in vitro fertilization. Fertil Steril 2008; 90:1662–1673.
7. Wang YA, Sullivan EA, Black D, et al. Preterm birth and low birth weight after assisted reproductive technology-related pregnancy in Australia between 1996 and 2000. Fertil Steril 2005; 83:1650–1658.
8. Malchau SS, Loft A, Larsen E, et al. Perinatal outcomes in 375 children born after oocyte donation: a Danish national cohort study. Fertil Steril 2013; 99:1637–1643.
9. Setti PEL, Albani E, Morenghi E, et al. Comparative analysis of fetal and neonatal outcomes of pregnancies from fresh and cryopreserved/thawed oocytes in the same group of patients. Fertil Steril 2013; 100:396–401.
10. Stucliffe A, Ludwig M. Outcome of assisted reproduction. Lancet 2007; 370:351–359.
11. Pehlivan T, Rubio C, Rodrigo L, et al. Impact of preimplantation genetic diagnosis on IVF outcome in implantation failure patients. Reprod Biomed Online 2003; 6:232–237.
12. Yang Z, Liu J, Collins GS, et al. Selection of single blastocysts for fresh transfer via standard morphology assessment alone and with array CGH for good prognosis IVF patients: results from a randomized pilot study. Mol Cytogenet 2012; 5:1–8.
13. Farhi Reichman B, Boyko V, Hourvitz A, et al. Maternal and neonatal health outcomes following assisted reproduction. Reprod Biomed Online 2013; 26:454–461.
14. Sazonova A, Kallen K, Thurin-Kjellberg A, et al. Obstetric outcome after in vitro fertilization with single or double embryo transfer. Hum Reprod 2011; 26:442–450.
15. Hayashi M, Nakai A, Satoh S, et al. Adverse obstetric and perinatal outcomes of singleton pregnancies may be related to maternal factors associated with infertility rather than the type of assisted reproductive technology procedure used. Fertil Steril 2012; 98:922–928.
16. Pecks U, Maass N, Neulen J. Oocyte donation: a risk factor for pregnancy-induced hypertension – a meta-analysis and case series. Dtsch Arztebl Int 2011; 108:23–31.

17. Bergh C, Wennerholm U. Obstetric outcome and long-term follow up of children conceived through assisted reproduction. Best Pract Res Clin Obstet Gynaecol 2012; 26:841–852.
18. Henningsen AA, Pinborg A. Birth and perinatal outcomes and complications of babies conceived following ART. Semin Fetal Neonatal Med 2014; 19:234–238.
19. Wang YA, Sullivan EA, Healy DL, et al. Perinatal outcomes after assisted reproductive technology treatment in Australia and New Zealand: single versus double embryo transfer. Med J Aust 2009; 190:234–237.
20. Sullivan EA, Chapman MG, Wang YA, et al. Population-based study of cesarean section after in-vitro fertilization in Australia. Birth 2010; 37:184–191.
21. Fauser BCJM, Devroey P, Diedrich K, et al. Annual Reproduction (EVAR) Workshop Group 2011. Health outcomes of children born after IVF/ICSI: a review of current expert opinion and literature. Reprod Biomed Online 2014; 28:162–182.
22. Davies MJ, Moore VM, Willson KJ, et al. Reproductive technologies and the risk of birth defects. N Engl J Med 2012; 366:1803–1813.
23. Zhu JL, Basso O, Obel C, et al. Infertility, infertility treatment and congenital malformations: Danish national birth cohort. BMJ 2006; 333:679.
24. Pinborg A, Henningsen AA, Malchau SS et al. Congenital anomalies after assisted reproductive technology. Fertil Steril 2013; 99:327–332.
25. Bay B, Mortensen EL, Kesmodel US. Assisted reproduction and child neurodevelopmental outcomes: a systematic review. Fertil Steril 2013; 100:844–853.
26. Kallen B. The risk of neurodisability and other long-term outcomes for infants born following ART. Semin Fetal Neonatal Med 2014; 19:239–244.
27. Hediger ML, Bell EM, Druschel CM, et al. Assisted reproductive technologies and children's neurodevelopmental outcomes. Fertil Steril 2013; 99:311–317.
28. Shankaran S. Outcomes from infancy to adulthood after assisted reproductive technology. Fertil Steril 2014; 101:1217–1221.
29. Yeung EH, Druschel C. Cardiometabolic health of children conceived by assisted reproductive technologies. Fertil Steril 2013; 99:318–326.
30. Rombauts L, Motteram C, Berkowitz E, et al. Risk of placenta praevia is linked to endometrial thickness in a retrospective cohort study of 4537 singleton assisted reproduction technology births. Hum Reprod 2014; 29(12):2787–2793.

Chapter 13

Induction of labour: who, when, how and where?

Kelly Mast, Mieke LG Ten Eikelder, Kitty WM Bloemenkamp,
Josje Langenveld, Ben Willem J Mol

INTRODUCTION

Induction of labour is one of the most used, and probably one of the most effective interventions in modern obstetrics. Globally, labour is induced in 20–30% of all deliveries, for a variety of reasons, amongst which hypertensive disorders in pregnancy, post-term pregnancy, intrauterine growth restriction (IUGR) and elective request are the most frequent [1–3]. The aim of induction of labour is to end the pregnancy, as continuation of the pregnancy could jeopardise the condition of the mother or her baby, and delivery is thought to be safer. The effectiveness of induction of labour can be evaluated by measuring the time taken to achieve a successful vaginal delivery, usually within a predefined time frame, e.g. 24 hours. Safety relates to good clinical condition of both mother and her baby.

Induction of labour was first described by Hippocrates, when he explained the effects of mammary stimulation and mechanical dilation of the cervical canal [4]. Although methods of inducing labour have been practised since then, the exact knowledge on whom, when, where and how to induce has been lacking. As with many interventions in modern medicine, there is no evidence-based consensus about who will really benefit from labour induction. More insight has, however, been provided by recent large, randomised controlled clinical trials (RCTs).

In this chapter, we describe four issues: how to induce labour; who needs induction; when is the optimal time and finally, where induction should take place.

RATIONALE FOR INDUCTION OF LABOUR

The decision for induction of labour is a balance between benefits and possible side effects in comparison to continuing the pregnancy. This decision, in keeping with many decisions

Kelly Mast MD, Department of Obstetrics and Gynaecology, Atrium Medisch Centrum Parkstad, The Netherlands. Email: cekmast@gmail.com (for correspondence)

Mieke LG Ten Eikelder MD, Department of Obstetrics, Leiden University Medical Center, Leiden, The Netherlands

Kitty WM Bloemenkamp MD PhD, Department of Obstetrics, Leiden University Medical Center, Leiden, The Netherlands

Josje Langenveld MD PhD, Department of Obstetrics and Gynaecology, Atrium Medical Centrum Parkstad, Heerlen, The Netherlands

Ben Willem J Mol MD PhD, The Robinson Institute, University of Adelaide, Adelaide, Australia

in obstetrics, has two dimensions: the dimension for the mother and the dimension for the child. The risks for the mother and child are related to continuing the pregnancy and to those of the induction process itself. For the child, there is the additional burden arising from the complications of prematurity. Thus, induction of labour is an intervention that should only be performed when the benefits of ending the pregnancy outweigh the benefits from continuation, either from the perspective of the mother, the child or both.

Maternal risks of continuing pregnancy arise when a woman has an underlying maternal disease exacerbated by pregnancy or where disease develops as a consequence of pregnancy, hypertension and pre-eclampsia being the most prominent examples. Delivery is the definitive cure for pregnancy-induced hypertension and pre-eclampsia such that early delivery by induction of labour can help prevent severe pregnancy complications such as eclampsia, stroke, liver rupture, haemorrhage from placental abruption and even death. For the child, continuation of pregnancy can bring additional risks including fetal growth restriction, traumatic delivery of large-for-gestational age babies in diabetic mothers and stillbirth, especially in post-term babies. Induction of labour on the other hand may jeopardise the well-being of the child because of the complications of prematurity.

A final issue in the balance between ending and continuing the pregnancy relates to the consequences of the induction procedure itself. Although it has long been thought that induction of labour is associated with an increase in the incidence of caesarean section, a recent meta-analysis showed no increase [5]. In general, induction of labour has no effect on the risk of caesarean section, but for the situation when continuation of pregnancy would increase the risk of a caesarean section. For example, in women with mild pre-eclampsia or pregnancy-induced hypertension, prolonging pregnancy is likely to result in deterioration of the mother and/or her baby's clinical condition such that induction of labour may reduce the rate of caesarean section. Women with an expected large-for-gestational baby might benefit from induction because further growth arising from expectant management may increase the likelihood of caesarean section. Induction of labour for fetal growth restriction does not affect the risk of caesarean section [6–8B].

The suggested increase in risk of caesarean section due to the induction of labour has been based on observational studies, comparing women in spontaneous labour to women in whom labour is induced [9]. However, the comparison of spontaneous labour to induced labour is not valid because in nonrandomised studies women with a worsening condition are induced, e.g. those who go on to be post-term, thereby selecting women who are more likely to have nonprogressive labour.

INDICATIONS FOR INDUCTION

Induction of labour is indicated for maternal or fetal reasons.

Fetal reasons

Intrauterine growth restriction

IUGR is associated with an increased risk of neonatal morbidity and stillbirth. Growth restriction implies a pathological limitation of the potential growth, likely caused by dysfunction of the placenta. As the diagnosis can only be suspected based on the assessment of fundal height or with ultrasound, suspected IUGR is defined as an estimated fetal weight (EFW) below the 10th percentile, fetal abdominal circumference below the

10th percentile, flattening of the growth curve in the third trimester or the presence of more than one of these factors [6].

The diagnosis of IUGR can be established by performing serial measurement of the symphysio-fundal height from 24 weeks of pregnancy. In cases of growth below the 10th percentile or suspected arrest of growth, ultrasound examination is recommended. For growth-restricted fetuses, evaluation of the umbilical artery blood flow Doppler should be considered [10]. The use of customised growth standards may differentiate pathologically as opposed to the physiologically small fetus. These growth curves are based on the fetus' growth potential [11].

Timing the delivery of a growth-restricted fetus has been subject of research. The Growth Restriction Intervention Trial (GRIT) included women with fetal compromise between 24 and 36 weeks and reported no differences between immediate delivery and expectant monitoring with respect to neonatal death or severe disability after 2 years [10% vs. 9%, odds ratio (OR) 1.1; 95% confidence interval (CI) 0.7–1.8]. Little contrast was seen between the immediate delivery and expectant management groups in terms of median time-to-delivery (0.9 days in the immediate group vs. 4.9 days in the delay group). Delivery can be considered when the fetus is ≥26 weeks, EFW is >500 g and lung maturation by corticosteroids has been completed. In these severe preterm cases, delivery by caesarean section is advised [10,32].

The Disproportionate Intrauterine Growth Intervention (DIGITAT) study was a randomised trial of comparing induction of labour and expectant management of 660 women with suspected IUGR fetuses at or near term (i.e. 36-40 weeks). A composite measure for adverse neonatal outcome occurred in 5.3% of fetuses in the induction group versus 6.1% in the expectant monitoring group (difference -0,8%; 95% CI -4.3 to 2.8). The caesarean section rate did not differ with a 14% incidence in both groups (difference 0.3%; 95% CI -5.0 to 5.6%) [6]. Thus, induction of labour did no harm in these women.

The optimal timing of delivery in the presence of IUGR is not easy to investigate prospectively. Epidemiological data, however, indicate that for women with a growth-restricted child, the cut-off where extrauterine survival is better than intrauterine survival appears to start at 38–39 weeks of gestation [12A]. Furthermore, in the DIGITAT study, the number of very small children, defined as below the 3rd percentile, delivered in women who were managed expectantly increased from 13% to 31% (difference 18.1%; 95% CI 12–24.3%; $P < 0.001$) indicating that expectant management may put these babies in jeopardy.

In practice, induction of labour will be recommended for most women with a growth-restricted fetus from 38 weeks of gestation to prevent possible neonatal morbidity. However, close expectant monitoring can be safely performed for the neonate according to the parent's wishes. Both induction and expectant management do not affect development and behavioural outcome in 2-year follow-up [12B]. When induction of labour is started, continuous fetal heart monitoring is recommended from the onset of contractions. Practitioners and parents should be aware of the higher rates of emergency caesarean section when the fetus is growth restricted [6].

Macrosomia

Macrosomia is defined as an estimated weight of at least 4000 g or a weight for gestational age >90th percentile, though multiple definitions are applied [8A]. Inducing labour where macrosomia is suspected has been practised because of fears about problematic delivery, in particular the risks for obstructed labour and shoulder dystocia. However, evidence supporting such an indication for prompting labour because of suspected fetal macrosomia in the absence of maternal diabetes is lacking with no risk reduction observed in terms of the likelihood of surgical or instrumental delivery, shoulder dystocia or birth injury. Indeed, a systematic review evaluating expectant management versus induction of labour in the presence of suspected fetal macrosomia suggested a lower risk of caesarean section in favour of allowing a spontaneous onset of labour (OR 0.39; 95% CI 0.30–0.50). The same review showed no risk reduction for shoulder dystocia by inducing labour (OR 0.93; 95% CI 0.35–2.46) [8A]. However, in contrast, a recent RCT showed a reduced risk for shoulder dystocia when induced compared to expectant management (RR 0,32, 95% CI 0,15-0,71; P=0,004) [8B].

These findings are based on small observational datasets, and the outcomes will be influenced by study characteristics such as the populations studied, diagnostic criteria and management of labour. In general, induction of labour should only be considered where there is strong evidence of a fetal weight above 4000 g or when attempting vaginal delivery after shoulder dystocia [13]. Sonography is more accurate in predicting EFW than clinical examination, but is still limited and lacks precision. If a decision is made to induce the labour because of suspected fetal macrosomia, the possibility of a prolonged induction time should be discussed with the prospective parents.

Diabetes

Induction of labour of a pregnancy that is complicated by diabetes is widely accepted. Major concerns in diabetic pregnancy involve stillbirth in the third trimester and macrosomia-related birth trauma. For women whose diabetes is medically managed by insulin or oral medicine, induction is recommended from 38 to 39 weeks of gestation. It lowers the chance of delivering a large baby, without increasing the risk of caesarean section [risk ratio (RR) 0.81; 95% CI 0.52–1.26] [14]. Earlier induction, with potential increase in fetal pulmonary complications and adverse maternal outcomes, in well regulated patients does not seem to be indicated. Caesarean delivery to reduce the risk of birth trauma can be considered where there is an EFW of >4500 g, but this remains debatable given the risks of surgical delivery because the number needed to treat to prevent one permanent brachial plexus injury is estimated to be 443 [15]. In the absence of large RCTs, clinical practice will vary amongst institutions.

Post-term pregnancy

Timely onset of labour and delivery is an important determinant of perinatal outcome. Both preterm and post-term births are associated with higher rates of perinatal morbidity and mortality compared with pregnancies delivering at term. Post-term pregnancy includes all pregnancies beyond 42 weeks' gestation or more precisely beyond 294 days, counted from the first day of the last menstrual period. In such pregnancies, the risk for stillbirth starts to increase considerably from 41 weeks onwards, although the absolute risk of neonatal death is low [16]. Other complications that occur more frequently after 41 weeks include meconium aspiration syndrome, oligohydramnios and fetal asphyxia. A Cochrane meta-analysis on this subject, including 16 studies, recommends induction of labour from 41 weeks in uncomplicated singleton pregnancies [16]. Since induction of labour might last several days, it might be considered at 41 weeks of gestation [17].

More recently, the benefits of elective induction of labour before 41 weeks' gestation have resurfaced in recognition that the risk of stillbirth begins to rise from 39 weeks onwards, especially in older women. A recent, small, single-centre RCT suggested that induction of labour at 39 weeks' gestation does not increase the risk of caesarean section (OR 0.92; 95% CI 0.76–1.12) [18] supporting previous data from some older studies [19]. However, the benefits of elective induction at 39 weeks need further study in the context of modern-day labour ward practices and to allow other neonatal and maternal outcomes to be accounted for. One such multicentre RCT (ARRIVE—https://clinicaltrials.gov/ct2/show/NCT01990612) is in progress comparing elective induction of labour at 39 weeks with expectant management in nulliparous women with singleton uncomplicated term pregnancies.

Preterm rupture of membranes

Induction of labour for prelabour rupture of the membranes at term is well accepted globally. However, expectant management appears safest in managing preterm rupture of the membranes. An RCT at late preterm (34–37 weeks) premature rupture of the membranes demonstrated no advantage in terms of the incidence of neonatal sepsis conferred by early induction as opposed to expectant management (3% vs. 4.1%; 95% CI 0.17–3.2). No other differences were observed for the secondary maternal or neonatal outcomes [20A]. In case of group B streptococcus vaginal contamination, induction of labor seems to be preferable as is reduces early onset neonatal sepsis from 15.2% to 1.8% [20B].

Cholestasis of pregnancy

Cholestasis is associated with preterm birth and has been thought to be associated with other complications in fetuses, such as stillbirth. Especially higher levels of bile acid (e.g. > 40 µmol/l during pregnancy) are thought to be associated with the risk of still birth, although there is little evidence to support these contentions. However, concerns over stillbirth and the difficulty to predict intrauterine fetal demise in the presence of obstetric cholestasis account for the policy of many obstetricians to electively induce labour preterm. Reporting on the management of cholestasis, 21 studies (1197 patients) were reviewed. However, timing of delivery was studied in solely one study with 63 patients, which showed no benefit in early delivery versus expectant management until 37 weeks of gestation. Therefore, there is still insufficient data to support preterm induction of labour. Medical treatment like ursodeoxycholic acid and S-adenosylmethionine can be started to reduce the symptoms of pruritus although not the potential risk of stillbirth [21].

Maternal reasons

Hypertension

Delivery of the placenta and as a consequence the baby is the only definite cure for women who develop hypertension in pregnancy. The decision for early delivery is influenced by the expected deterioration in either the maternal or fetal condition from the pregnancy continuing.

The first HYPITAT RCT compared induction of labour with expectant monitoring for gestational hypertension or mild pre-eclampsia after 36 weeks' gestation. The study showed that induction of labour leads to a decrease in progression to severe disease or maternal complications as compared to expectant management (31% vs. 44%; RR 0.71; 95% CI 0.59–0.86; $P < 0.001$), without increasing the caesarean section rate. The HYPITAT study has subsequently been criticised for selecting a composite primary outcome that included occurrence of severe hypertension in addition to the more serious complications of pre-eclampsia such as eclampsia and HELLP syndrome (haemolysis, elevated liver enzymes, low platelet count). Although one can argue whether this composite outcome is really homogeneous, the study supports induction from 39 weeks onwards for all women with hypertension in pregnancy and from 37 weeks in women with pre-eclampsia [7].

Whether women with mild preeclampsia or severe hypertension between 34 and 37 weeks should be offered induction of labour was the subject of the HYPITAT II study. This randomised trial showed no differences in maternal outcome, but there was significantly more respiratory distress syndrome amongst the neonates in the immediate delivery group [22]. Based on the findings from this RCT study, routine induction of labour for the indication of mild pre-eclampsia or severe hypertension before 37 weeks cannot be recommended. However, the mother should be well monitored in this period. In contrast, women who develop severe pre-eclampsia or HELLP syndrome between 34 and 37 weeks should be delivered after the administration of corticosteroids for fetal lung maturity if before 34 weeks' gestation [22–24].

Previous caesarean section

Globally, the caesarean section rate is rising (most are significantly over 15%) [25A], with an increase in maternal and neonatal morbidity and mortality. The optimal caesarean section rate is under review by the World Health Organisation [25B]. One of the reasons for the observed increase in morbidity and mortality is the rising incidence of uterine ruptures associated with subsequent attempted vaginal deliveries. Rupture of the uterine wall, i.e. disruption or tearing of the uterine muscle and visceral peritoneum, with or without extension into the bladder or broad ligament, is considered a severe complication. Elective, repeat caesarean sections are not devoid of risk and vaginal delivery after previous low transverse caesarean section is an option and the advantages and disadvantages of vaginal or elective caesarean delivery should be discussed with the woman. A large, well-designed prospective study reported an absolute risk of uterine rupture during attempted vaginal delivery after previous caesarean section of 1% with induction of labour versus 0.4% with spontaneous labour (OR 2.86; 95% CI 1.75–4.67) [26]. Many variables appear to affect this risk, e.g. augmentation with oxytocin, the favourability of the cervix prior to induction and the method of induction itself. In a population-based, retrospective cohort analysis, uterine rupture was more likely amongst women with spontaneous onset of labour (RR 3.3; 95% CI 1.8–6.0), induction of labour without prostaglandins (RR 4.9; 95% CI 2.4–9.7) and induction with prostaglandins (RR 15.6; 95% CI 8.1–30.0) compared with the risk in women with repeated elective caesarean delivery.

Thus, induction of labour with oxytocin or prostaglandins in women with a previous caesarean section requires careful consideration. Close monitoring is required and steps should be taken to minimise the risks of uterine hyperstimulation.

Maternal age

In the near future, we will probably consider this indication more frequently as women are increasingly delaying childbirth. Increasing maternal age is related with more co-morbidity and obstetric complications such as pre-eclampsia and gestational diabetes. Controlled for these pre-existing maternal conditions, maternal age is still found as an independent risk for delivery-related perinatal death at term [27]. Absolute risk seems to be low, but induction at 39 weeks might just improve neonatal outcome based on the finding that risk of stillbirth is equal for women aged >40 years at gestation of 39 weeks compared to mothers aged 25–29 years at gestation of 41 weeks [28], suggesting a benefit in inducing woman with advanced age.

Whether induction of labour indeed will reduce the risk of stillbirth and other obstetric complications needs further research. The 35/39-Trial studies the risk of caesarean section when induced at 39 weeks compared to expectant management in women over 35 years of age. The study is currently recruiting (www.controlled-trials.com/ISRCTN11517275/).

Maternal request

Social reasons for induction of labour at term are perhaps the most contentious. Induction of labour on request remains debatable mostly because of the increased risks for surgical delivery. The counterargument is that these risks may be minimised with careful counselling and management of labour. This includes informing the woman of the possibility of a prolonged induction process >24 hours to achieve a vaginal delivery providing providing both mother and baby are in good condition. There is growing evidence that induction of labour does not increase surgical delivery or other complications [29,30].

WHEN TO INDUCE

We have discussed in the preceding sections the reasons to wait for induction of labour until gestation has reached term. Not infrequently, however, we are confronted with the dilemma of ending the pregnancy preterm. Preterm pregnancy describes delivery of the fetus before 37 weeks of gestation. In the preterm period, we can differentiate early preterm delivery (before 34 weeks of gestation) and late preterm delivery (described as 34–37 weeks of gestation). Infants born early preterm, when born alive, are exposed to many risks. Respiratory distress, patent ductus arteriosus, intraventricular haemorrhage, late-onset sepsis and bronchopulmonary dysplasia are frequently occurring neonatal morbidities in this period. Administration of corticosteroids significantly reduces the risk for intraventricular haemorrhage (RR 0.54), necrotising enterocolitis (RR 0.46), neonatal mortality (RR 0.69) and systemic infection in the first 48 hours of life (RR 0.56) and should be given to all women with likely risk of early premature birth [31].

Severe pre-eclampsia or HELLP syndrome, suspected infection after rupture of the membranes or fetal compromise are common indications for preterm induction of labour. When gestational age is early preterm, often a surgical delivery cannot be avoided, due to condition of mother and/or fetus. Decision making in these cases should be individualised and within an experienced, multidisciplinary obstetric team. In late preterm gestation, induction of labour should be delayed until 37 weeks or until deterioration in the condition of mother or child. Several seminal trials such as DIGITAT [6,10], HYPITAT-II [24] and PROMEXILL [20A] supported delay of induction of labour until term period.

Thus, preterm induction of labour should be considered carefully and the relative risks of ending the pregnancy compared to continuing in the current situation judiciously evaluated. In many cases, the decision for delivery should be re-evaluated on a daily basis.

HOW TO INDUCE

The method of inducing labour should be based on both effectiveness and safety, i.e. the baby is delivered within the time that is set for the induction and in a good condition. Clinical studies have often selected time to delivery as their main endpoint, but the combination of effectiveness should be considered in tandem. As Dwight Rouse stated in a recent commentary: 'Driving 100 miles per hour may get you home from work a bit earlier, but is usually not a good idea' [33].

During pregnancy, the cervix serves as 'the gatekeeper' of the uterus. It forms a barrier for bacteria and helps maintain the physical integrity of the uterus for the benefit of fetal development until delivery. When labour starts, the cervix starts to soften and efface, a process called cervical ripening. Cytokines, nitric oxide synthesis, enzymes, prostaglandins and hormones are integral to this process. Cervical ripening represents the beginning of the first stage of labour, the so-called 'latent phase' and some dilatation of the cervix might occur. The 'active phase' is recognised when regular, strong uterine contractions establish which lead to progressive dilatation of the cervix until full dilatation is attained. The active stage of the first stage of labour takes 7.7 hours for nulliparous women and 5.6 hours for multiparous women on average (statistical limits of two standard deviations from the mean are 17.5 and 13.8 hours, respectively) [34].

The choice of method for induction of labour depends on the ripeness of the cervix. Cervical assessment includes a digital vaginal examination with evaluation of cervical dilatation, effacement, position, consistency and the fetal station in the pelvis. Bishop described a prelabour scoring system using these five components [35]. Scores of <6 generally require that a cervical ripening method should be used before other methods.

Mechanical methods

Membrane sweeping

'Sweeping' the membranes can be used to reduce the need of a formal induction with prostaglandins or oxytocin [35]. The technique of 'stripping' or 'sweeping' the membranes is simple: during vaginal examination, the finger is introduced into the cervical canal, and by moving the finger in a circular motion, the membranes become separated from the lower uterine segment. This precipitates local production of prostaglandins by the induction of phospholipase A2 in the cervical and membrane tissues. Sweeping the membranes is not related to an increased risk of caesarean section, asphyxia or other fetal or maternal morbidity or mortality [35]. No major maternal side effects have been reported, but pain during vaginal examination and blood loss occur frequently. To avoid one formal induction of labour at term, eight women need membrane sweeping from 38 weeks pregnancy onwards [35]. Therefore, it is a workable method in nonurgent indications for induction of labour and is suitable as an outpatient procedure.

Amniotomy

The aim of artificial rupture of the membranes is to strengthen uterine contractions to accelerate labour. Puncturing the membranes, i.e. the amnion and chorion with an amnihook to release the amniotic fluid is thought to initiate labour by triggering the release of prostaglandins and oxytocin, inducing and enforcing uterine contractions. Associated risks with amniotomy include cord prolapse and malpresentation of the fetus, especially in the presence of polyhydramnios, prematurity or when the fetal presenting part is not engaged. Vasa praevia, where fetal vessels run within the membranes, is a rare contraindication to amniotomy. The condition cannot always be detected antenatally and the possibility of vasa praevia should be considered in the presence of painless bleeding associated with changes in fetal heart rate following amniotomy.

Balloon

Dilation of the cervix using balloon devices has been practised for over a century. Until the 1940s, the 'meteurynter', a conic bag that was placed beyond the cervix and filled with saline solution, was the instrument of choice for dilation of the cervix. Treub first used the urinary catheter in 1890, although the balloon was then filled up to 500 mL of saline in contrast to the much smaller fluid volumes from 30 to 80 mL used today [36].

The working mechanism of transcervical placement of a Foley catheter is not solely mechanical. Its effect in inducing ripening and dilation is also achieved by increasing local prostaglandin production [37]. The catheter is inserted and placed just beyond the internal cervical os and the balloon is filled with saline. Traction may be applied in addition. More adaptations of the catheter are currently available. The Atad balloon or double balloon catheter is similarly inserted, both supracervical and cervicovaginal balloons which can be inflated up to 100 mL [38]. Both Foley and Atad catheters are related to a longer induction to delivery interval compared to pharmacological agents, but they were associated with less uterine hyperstimulation and similar caesarean section rates. Concurrent extra-amniotic saline infusion (EASI) instilled through a transcervical Foley catheter may increase successful vaginal delivery compared to any vaginal prostaglandin and the rate of uterine hyperstimulation with fetal heart changes appears to be similar. Furthermore, the risk of caesarean section was not statistically increased in the EASI group compared with prostaglandins (32% vs. 22%). Maternal and neonatal morbidity was also low [39]. Compared to the use of PGE2 gel (dinoprostone), the Foley catheter has comparable induction to delivery duration and caesarean section rates with less maternal and neonatal morbidity [42A, 42B]. When compared to vaginal application of misoprostol, induction by Foley catheter is associated with reduced uterine hyperstimulation causing adverse fetal heart changes [42C].

Pharmacological methods

Prostaglandins

In obstetrics, prostaglandines, synthesised from polyunsaturated fatty acids, made their introduction in the late 1960s. Their exact mechanism of action has yet to be elucidated. It is thought that prostaglandins may cause a higher production of hyaluronic acid by the cervical fibroblast, resulting in an increase in water molecules intercalating amongst the collagen fibres [40A]. A complex process of re-alignment of collagen, degradation of collagen-crosslinking in combination with uterine contractions results in cervical dilation. Prostaglandin receptors are found in the cervix as well as the myometrium. Prostaglandins induce uterine contractions and cervical ripening which often results in the onset of labour without the need for additional methods such as amniotomy and oxytocin. Identification of the first stage of labour can therefore be more difficult. The most commonly used prostaglandins are PGE_1 and PGE_2. Routes of administration studied have included oral, sublingual and buccal, but the most common route of administration is vaginal using tablets, suppositories, gels and pessaries.

Misoprostol

Misoprostol, a derivative of PGE_1, is being widely used in pregnant women for cervical ripening and induction of labour. Originally, misoprostol was prescribed for the treatment of gastric ulcers and is still not registered for obstetrical use and as such constitutes an 'off label' prescription. In spite of that, misoprostol has been proven highly effective in termination of pregnancy in the first or second trimester and has been used effectively for cervical ripening and induction of labour at term.

Misoprostol is given as a tablet and taken either orally or vaginally. Peak plasma levels are reached more rapidly when taken orally (34±17 min) than vaginally (80±27 min). This might be due to the first-pass effect that occurs with oral application. Oral administration results in a shorter activity period [40A].

Misoprostol can be administered in different dosages and regimes. Most often, a maximum daily dose of 150 µg is used. Both oral and vaginal administration of misoprostol appear to be more effective than other prostaglandins, that is in achieving vaginal delivery within 24 hours of induction vaginal misoprostol tablets (>50ug) are the most effective and oral misoprostol titrated in low dose (<50ug) has the lowest probability of caesarean section [41A]. Furthermore, the use of misoprostol is associated with fewer caesarean sections compared with vaginal dinoprostone (RR 0,88, 95% CI 0,78 to 0,99) or oxytocin (RR 0,77, 95% CI 0,60 to 0,98) without risks of adverse maternal and perinatal outcomes [41B]. However, uterine hyperstimulation with nonreassuring fetal heart rate changes might be more prevalent with vaginal application of misoprostol compared with the oral route. However, this observed effect may be dose related [41A,42B]. Compared with higher doses of vaginal misoprostol, lower doses were associated with a reduced risk of hyperstimulation [41B]. Other benefits of misoprostol compared to vaginal dinoprostone include the low cost of misoprostol and the possibility of storing the tablets at room temperature.

Oxytocin

Induction of labour using only oxytocin (without ruptured membranes) does not seem to be effective as a method of induction. Compared with vaginal prostaglandins, oxytocin increased unsuccessful vaginal delivery within 24 hours in the two trials reporting this outcome (70% versus 21%, RR 3.33, 95% CI 1.61 to 6.89) as well as increasing the likelihood of requiring epidural anaesthesia (RR 1.09, 95% CI 1.01 to 1.17) [40B]. When membranes are ruptured however, augmentation with the use of intravenous oxytocin reduces the likelihood of not delivering within 24 hours (RR 0.03, 95% CI 0.001-0.49). Furthermore augmenting with oxytocin results in significantly fewer instrumental vaginal deliveries compared with placebo (RR 0.18, CI 0.05-0.58) [43].

WHERE TO INDUCE

Hospital delivery is commonplace in the developed world where induction of labour is required. However, considering the safety of different methods of cervical ripening, there might be a place for induction in an outpatient setting. Several potential benefits could be gained by cervical ripening in a nonclinical situation including less time spent in hospital, higher patient satisfaction and lower costs [44]. Large-scale trials are needed to evaluate the efficacy and safety of home versus hospital settings for induction of labour and to identify which patient groups would benefit most.

Key points for clinical practice

- Induction of labour is one of the most effective interventions in obstetric care. When timed properly, it can prevent serious complications for mother and child, with little additional risk for the neonate and without an increased risk of caesarean section.

- For many indications, evidence for the optimal timing of induction has been elucidated preferring timing at term. When preterm induction is considered it should offer maternal and/or fetal benefits.

- In case of an unripe cervix, mechanical induction with transcervical balloon and oral misoprostol are probably the safest methods.

- When induction of labour is started, the condition of both mother and child should be the indicator for further decision making instead of induction time.

REFERENCES

1. Zeitlin J, Mohangoo A, Delnord M, et al. European Perinatal Health Report. The health and care of pregnant women and babies in Europe in 2010. Paris; European Perinatal Health, 2013.
2. National Health Service (NHS). NHS Maternity Statistics––England, 2012-13. London; NHS, 2013.
3. Martin JA, Hamilton BE, Osterman MJK, et al. Births: Final Data for 2012. National Vital Statistics Reports 2013; 62.
4. de Ribes C. De l'Accouchement Provoque, Dilatation du Canal Genital a l'Aide de Ballons Introduits dans la Cavite Uterine Pendant la Grossesse. Paris: Steinheil; 1988.
5. Wood S, Cooper S, Ross S. Does induction of labour increase the risk of caesarean section? A systematic review and meta-analysis of trials in women with intact membranes. BJOG 2014; 121:674–685; discussion 85.
6. Boers KE, Vijgen SM, Bijlenga D, et al. Induction versus expectant monitoring for intrauterine growth restriction at term: randomised equivalence trial (DIGITAT). BMJ 2010; 341:c7087.
7. Koopmans CM, Bijlenga D, Groen H, et al. Induction of labour versus expectant monitoring for gestational hypertension or mild pre-eclampsia after 36 weeks' gestation (HYPITAT): a multicentre, open-label randomised controlled trial. Lancet 2009; 374:979–988.
8A. Sanchez-Ramos L, Bernstein S, Kaunitz AM. Expectant management versus labor induction for suspected fetal macrosomia: a systematic review. Obstet Gynecol 2002; 100:997–1002.
8B. 8B - Boulvain M, Senat MV, Perrotin F, et al. Groupe de Recherche en Obstétrique et Gynécologie (GROG). Induction of labour versus expectant management for large-for-date fetuses: a randomised controlled trial. Lancet 2015 Apr 8. pii: S0140-6736(14)61904-8.
9. Vrouenraets FP, Roumen FJ, Dehing CJ, et al. Bishop score and risk of cesarean delivery after induction of labor in nulliparous women. Obstet Gynecol 2005; 105:690–697.
10. RCOG. Small-for-gestational-age fetus, investigation and management (Green-top 31). Royal College of Obstetricians and Gynaecologists, 2013.
11. Clausson B, Gardosi J, Francis A, et al. Perinatal outcome in SGA births defined by customised versus population-based birthweight standards. BJOG 2001; 108:830–834.
12A. Kazemier BM, Voskamp BJ, Ravelli AC, et al. Optimal timing of delivery in small for gestational age fetuses near term: a national cohort study. Am J Perinatol 2015; 30:177–186.
12B. an Wyk L, Boers KE, van der Post JA, et al. DIGITAT Study Group. Effects on (neuro)developmental and behavioral outcome at 2 years of age of induced labor compared with expectant management in intrauterine growth-restricted infants: long-term outcomes of the DIGITAT trial. Am J Obstet Gynecol 2012; 206):406.e1-7.
13. Boulvain M, Senat M-V, Rozenberg P, et al. Induction of labor or expectant management for large-for-dates fetuses: a randomized controlled trial. Am J Obstet Gynecol 2012; 206:S2.

14. Boulvain M, Stan Catalin M, Irion O. Elective delivery in diabetic pregnant women. Cochrane Database Syst Rev. 2001; (2):CD001997.
15. Rouse DJ, Owen J, Goldenberg RL, et al. The effectiveness and costs of elective cesarean delivery for fetal macrosomia diagnosed by ultrasound. JAMA 1996; 276:1480–1486.
16. Sanchez-Ramos L, Olivier F, Delke I, et al. Labor induction versus expectant management for postterm pregnancies: a systematic review with meta-analysis (structured abstract). Obstet Gynecol 2003; 101:1312–1318.
17. Hilder L, Costeloe K, Thilaganathan B. Prolonged pregnancy: evaluating gestation-specific risks of fetal and infant mortality. Br J Obstet Gynaecol 1998; 105:169–173.
18. Miller NR, Cypher RL, Foglia LM, et al. Elective induction of nulliparous labor at 39 weeks of gestation: a randomized clinical trial. Obstet Gynecol 2014; 123 Suppl 1:72S.
19. Caughey AB, Sundaram V, Kaimal AJ, et al. Maternal and neonatal outcomes of elective induction of labor. Evid Rep Technol Assess (Full Rep) 2009; (176):1–257.
20A. van der Ham DP, van der Heyden JL, Opmeer BC, et al. Management of late-preterm premature rupture of membranes: the PPROMEXIL-2 trial. Am J Obstet Gynecol 2012; 207:276.e1–276.e10.
20B. Tajik P, van der Ham DP, Zafarmand MH, et al. Using vaginal Group B Streptococcus colonisation in women with preterm premature rupture of membranes to guide the decision for immediate delivery: a secondary analysis of the PPROMEXIL trials. BJOG 2014; 121:1263-73.
21. Gurung V, Stokes M, Middleton P, et al. Interventions for treating cholestasis in pregnancy. Cochrane Database Syst Rev 2013; (6):CD000493.
22. Broekhuijsen K, van Baaren GJ, van Pampus MG, et al. HYPITAT-II study group. Immediate delivery versus expectant monitoring for hypertensive disorders of pregnancy between 34 and 37 weeks of gestation (HYPITAT-II): an open-label, randomised controlled trial. Lancet 2015 Mar 24. pii: S0140-6736(14)61998-X.
23. National Institute of Health and Clinical Excellence (NICE. Hypertension in pregnancy: the management of hypertensive disorders during pregnancy, clinical guideline, no. 107. London; NICE, 2010.
24. Langenveld J, Broekhuijsen K, van Baaren GJ, et al. Induction of labour versus expectant monitoring for gestational hypertension or mild pre-eclampsia between 34 and 37 weeks' gestation (HYPITAT-II): a multicentre, open-label randomised controlled trial. BMC Pregnancy Childbirth 2011; 11:50.
25A. Gibbons L, Belizan J, Lauer J, et al. The global numbers and costs of additionally needed and unnecessary caesarean sections performed per year: overuse as a barrier to universal coverage. World Health Report. Geneva, Switzerland: World Health Organization; 2010.
25B. World health organization (WHO). WHO statement n caesarean section rates. Executive summary. Geneva, WHO, 2015.
26. Landon MB, Hauth JC, Leveno KJ, et al. Maternal and perinatal outcomes associated with a trial of labor after prior cesarean delivery. N Engl J Med 2004; 351:2581–2589.
27. Gilbert WM, Nesbitt TS, Danielsen B. Childbearing beyond age 40: pregnancy outcome in 24,032 cases. Obstet Gynecol 1999; 93:9–14.
28. Reddy UM, Ko CW, Willinger M. Maternal age and the risk of stillbirth throughout pregnancy in the United States. Am J Obstet Gynecol 2006; 195:764–770.
29. Bircher C, Shepstone L, Yushchenko I, et al. Induction of labour for maternal request: An observational study of maternal and fetal outcomes. Rev Recent Clin Trials 2014 Aug 24 [Epub ahead of print].
30. Stock SJ, Ferguson E, Duffy A, et al. Outcomes of elective induction of labour compared with expectant management: population based study. BMJ 2012; 344:e2838.
31. Roberts D, Dalziel S. Antenatal corticosteroids for accelerating fetal lung maturation for women at risk of preterm birth. Cochrane Database Syst Rev 2006; (3):CD004454.
32. GRIT Group Study. A randomised trial of timed delivery for the compromised preterm fetus: short term outcomes and Bayesian interpretation. BJOG 2003; 110:27–32.
33. Rouse DJ. The misoprostol vaginal insert: deja vu all over again. Obstet Gynecol 2013; 122:193–194.
34. Albers LL. The duration of labor in healthy women. J Perinatol 1999; 19:114–119.
35. GRIT Group Study. GRIT Group Study.
36. Keirse M. Het inleiden van de baring - een eeuwenoude strijd voor heerschappij over de zwangerschapsduur. Obstetrische interventies - Geschiedenis en technieken. Medicom Europe B.V.; 1991:115-133
37. Manabe Y, Okazaki T, Takahashi A. Prostaglandins E and F in amniotic fluid during stretch-induced cervical softening and labor at term. Gynecol Obstet Invest 1983; 15:343–350.
38. Atad J, Hallak M, Auslender R, et al. A randomized comparison of prostaglandin E2, oxytocin, and the double-balloon device in inducing labor. Obstet Gynaecol 1996; 87:223-7.

39. Jozwiak M, Bloemenkamp KW, Kelly AJ, et al. Mechanical methods for induction of labour. Cochrane Database Syst Rev 2012; 3:CD001233.

40A. Arias F. Pharmacology of oxytocin and prostaglandins. Clin Obstet Gynecol 2000; 43:455–468.

40B. Alfirevic Z, Kelly Anthony J, Dowswell T. Intravenous oxytocin alone for cervical ripening and induction of labour. Cochrane Database Syst Rev 2009; 4:CD003246.

41A. Alfirevic Z, Keeney E, Dowswell T, et al. Labour induction with prostaglandins: a systematic review and network meta-analysis. BMJ 2015; 350:217.

41B. Alfirevic Z, Aflaifel N, Weeks A. Oral misoprostol for induction of labour. Cochrane Database Syst Rev 2014; 6:CD001338.

41C. Hofmeyr GJ, Gülmezoglu AM, Pileggi C. Vaginal misoprostol for cervical ripening and induction of labour. Cochrane Database Syst Rev 2010; (10).

42A. Jozwiak M, Oude Rengerink K, Benthem M, et al. Foley catheter versus vaginal prostaglandin E2 gel for induction of labour at term (PROBAAT trial): an open-label, randomised controlled trial. Lancet 2011; 378:2095–2103.

42B. World Health Organization (WHO), Department of Reproductive Health and Research. WHO recommendations for induction of labour. Geneva: WHO, 2011.

42C. Jozwiak M, ten Eikelder M, Oude Rengerink K, et al. Foley catheter versus vaginal misoprostol: randomized controlled trial (PROBAAT-M study) and systematic review and meta-analysis of literature. Am J Perinatol 2014; 31:145-56.

43. Howarth G, Botha Danie J. Amniotomy plus intravenous oxytocin for induction of labour. Cochrane Database Syst Rev. 2001; 3::CD003250.

44. Sciscione AC, Bedder CL, Hoffman MK, et al. The timing of adverse events with Foley catheter preinduction cervical ripening; implications for outpatient use. Am J Perinatol 2014; 31:781–786.

Index

Note: Page numbers in **bold** or *italic* refer to tables or figures, respectively.